Liver Diseases in the Pediatric Intensive Care Unit

Philippe Jouvet • Fernando Alvarez
Editors

Liver Diseases in the Pediatric Intensive Care Unit

A Clinical Guide

Springer

Editors
Philippe Jouvet
Pediatric Intensive Care Unit - Department of Pediatrics of Sainte Justine Hospital
University of Montreal
Montréal, QC
Canada

Fernando Alvarez
Division of Gastroenterology
Hepatology & Nutrition
Department of Pediatrics of Sainte Justine Hospital, University of Montreal
Montréal, QC
Canada

ISBN 978-3-030-79131-5 ISBN 978-3-030-79132-2 (eBook)
https://doi.org/10.1007/978-3-030-79132-2

This Springer imprint is published by the registered company Springer Nature Switzerland AG
The registered company address is: Gewerbestrasse 11, 6330 Cham, Switzerland

To the children with liver diseases, their families, and the caregivers who take care of them

Preface

For several years, we have observed an increase in liver damage in children hospitalized in the pediatric intensive care unit (PICU) of our institution. In many cases, this increase is due to the application and expansion of new technologies or therapeutic strategies, in others it is the consequence of intensive treatments administered in order to allow patients to have access to liver transplantation. Sometimes the liver "suffers in silence," and in such circumstances, this can initiate a sequence of events leading to multi-organ failure. Early diagnosis of liver injury from many different causes could prevent further deterioration. In addition, precise control of the increase in the number of drugs prescribed in PICU could prevent permanent toxic damage or establish a close monitoring.

The main objective of this book is to gather as much experience as possible in one volume, and to identify gaps in our knowledge in order to motivate clinical studies and basic research, with the aim of implementing continuous improvement in the management of children with primary or secondary liver diseases in PICU. The high damage tolerance and regenerative capacities of the liver tissue must be protected and supported to allow full recovery from acute or more or less chronic damage. Assessing the possibility of restoration of normal liver function after severe liver injury is a difficult and, in some cases, impossible task, leading to organ replacement. We need new reliable markers to better avoid liver transplantation in case of possible recovery and to better select children who can benefit from liver regeneration treatments that may appear in the future. In most of the chapters of this book, we associated young with experienced physicians, trying to make them aware of the prevention and early treatment of liver complications, and encouraging their involvement in the analysis and research of new diagnostic tools and therapeutic options.

Another relevant feature of this book is related to the interdisciplinary effort necessary for the care of children in the PICU, and the involvement of many professionals and scientists in order to offer the "best available options to our patients." In this sense, we are thinking of incorporating new chapters in the next edition, such as pharmacology and toxicity or nutrition and liver. Research is being developed on these topics in our institution. We also hope that this publication will expand collaborations and networks, thus accelerating new discoveries to improve quality of care.

We would like to thank all the colleagues who participated in this publication, for their openness during several fruitful discussions, and for their valuable support for this work. We would also like to acknowledge the invaluable trust conferred to us by the children and their families, which makes our daily task rewarding and motivates us to seek original alternatives to help them in such difficult situations.

Montréal, QC, Canada

Fernando Alvarez
Philippe Jouvet

Contents

Contributors

Fernando Alvarez, MD Division of Gastroenterology, Hepatology & Nutrition, Department of Pediatrics of Sainte Justine Hospital, University of Montreal, Montréal, QC, Canada

Sylvain Balandier, MD Pediatric Intensive Care Unit, Department of Pediatrics, CHU Sainte-Justine, Université de Montréal, Montreal, QC, Canada

Lucile Barcat, MD Pediatric Intensive Care Unit, Department of Pediatrics, CHU Sainte-Justine, Université de Montréal, Montreal, QC, Canada

Marie-Eve Chartier, MD Division of Gastroenterology, Hepatology and Nutrition, CHU Sainte-Justine, Université de Montréal, Montreal, QC, Canada

Laurence Ducharme Crevier, MD, MSc Pediatric Intensive Care Unit, Department of Pediatrics, CHU Sainte-Justine, Université de Montréal, Montreal, QC, Canada

Karen Harrington, MD, MSc Pediatric Intensive Care Unit, Department of Pediatrics, CHU Sainte-Justine, Université de Montréal, Montreal, QC, Canada

Philippe Jouvet, MD, PhD Pediatric Intensive Care Unit - Department of Pediatrics of Sainte Justine Hospital, University of Montreal, Montréal, QC, Canada

Jean-Sébastien Joyal, MD, PhD Pediatric Intensive Care Unit, Department of Pediatrics, CHU Sainte-Justine, Université de Montréal, Montreal, QC, Canada

Atsushi Kawaguchi, MD, PhD Pediatric Intensive Care Unit - Department of Pediatrics, CHU Sainte-Justine, University of Montreal, Montreal, QC, Canada

Department of Intensive Care Medicine, Tokyo Women's Medical University, Tokyo, Japan

Annie Lavoie, Pharmacist Department of Pharmacist, CHU Sainte-Justine, Université de Montréal, Montreal, QC, Canada

Massimiliano Paganelli, MD, PhD Pediatric Hepatology, CHU Sainte-Justine, Université de Montréal, Montreal, QC, Canada

Liver Tissue Engineering and Cell Therapy Laboratory, CHU Sainte-Justine Research Center, Montreal, QC, Canada

Virginie Plante, MD Pediatric Intensive Care Unit, Department of Pediatrics, CHU Sainte-Justine, Université de Montréal, Montreal, QC, Canada

Jean-Philippe Roy, MD Nephrology Unit, Department of Pediatrics, CHU Sainte-Justine, University of Montreal, Montreal, QC, Canada

Laurence Tabone, MD, MSc Pediatric Intensive Care Unit, Department of Pediatrics, CHU Sainte-Justine, Université de Montréal, Montreal, QC, Canada

Pierre Teira, MD, MSc Hematology-Oncology Unit, Department of Pediatrics, CHU Sainte-Justine, Université de Montréal, Montreal, QC, Canada

Genevieve Du Pont Thibodeau, MD, MSc Pediatric Intensive Care Unit, Department of Pediatrics, CHU Sainte-Justine, Université de Montréal, Montreal, QC, Canada

Liver Injury and Failure in Critically Ill Children

Virginie Plante and Philippe Jouvet

In critically ill patients, various insults can lead to secondary liver injury. Hepatic dysfunction is frequent in the intensive care unit and its occurrence is known to be associated with poorer outcomes. However, its diagnostic remains a challenge, mainly because of the lack of specificity of current markers and because of multiples confounders in complex critically ill patients. This chapter will review the pathophysiology, classification and care of liver injury and failure in critically ill children without pre-existing hepatobiliary disease.

Epidemiology

Abnormal liver tests are a frequent event in the intensive care unit. Thompson et al. [1] reported a prevalence as high as 61% at intensive care unit (ICU) admission in an adult population. Overt cholestasis (with definitions varying from a total bilirubin level greater than 34 µmol/L to 51 µmol/L) is found in 11–20% of critically ill adults [2–4]. It is even more common in certain subgroups of ICU patients, with a prevalence of up to 33% in septic shock and 21% in cardiogenic shock [4]. As for hepatocellular injury, the prevalence of hypoxic liver injury (defined as aminotransferase levels >5–20 folds above normal depending on studies) ranges between 1.5% and 4% in recent large adult ICU series [5–7].

V. Plante
Pediatric Intensive Care Unit, Department of Pediatrics, CHU Sainte-Justine, Université de Montréal, Montreal, QC, Canada
e-mail: virginie.plante.med1@ssss.gouv.qc.ca

P. Jouvet (✉)
Pediatric Intensive Care Unit - Department of Pediatrics of Sainte Justine Hospital, University of Montreal, Montréal, QC, Canada
e-mail: philippe.jouvet.med@ssss.gouv.qc.ca

P. Jouvet, F. Alvarez (eds.), *Liver Diseases in the Pediatric Intensive Care Unit*,
https://doi.org/10.1007/978-3-030-79132-2_1

Pediatric data on the prevalence of acquired liver injury in critically ill children is scarce, but abnormal liver testing at PICU admission is a common occurrence [8]. Jenniskens et al. [9] showed that while overt liver injury seems to be less frequent than in adult ICUs, it is still a significant problem, with a prevalence of almost 5% for cholestasis and 2% for hypoxic hepatitis. In children admitted after cardiac surgery, it is even more common, with 12% of patients presenting elevated transaminases and up to 4.7% with aminotransferase levels >20 folds above normal [10].

Cholestasis and hypoxic liver injury are a significant problem in critically ill children especially after cardiac surgery.

While hepatic injury was traditionally viewed as a late organ dysfunction, it is now known that early liver dysfunction is a strong and independent predictor of ICU mortality [2, 4, 5, 11, 12]. In adults, it is also associated with an increased length of stay and with the development of renal failure and secondary infections. The reported mortality rate in critically ill adults with acquired cholestasis is as high as 23% to 57% [2, 4, 5]. Abnormal liver tests are also associated with increased mortality in pediatric patients [9, 10]. Interestingly, the relationship between day 1 total bilirubin levels and mortality was found to be U-shaped in children, with levels below 3.4 μmol/L and above 13 μmol/L associated with increased mortality independently of baseline factors and severity of illness [9]. This raises the question of a possible protective effect of mild elevations of bilirubin that is hypothesized to be linked to an anti-inflammatory effect [13, 14].

Hepatic dysfunction has been included in multiple ICU prognostic scoring algorithms (Table 1), including the Pediatric Sequential Organ Failure Assessment Score (pSOFA) and the Pediatric Multiple Organ Dysfunction Score (P-MODS).

Pathophysiology of Liver Injury in Critically Ill Patients

Multiple factors can contribute to secondary liver injury in ICU patients. The pathophysiology is complex as there is often more than one mechanism in cause in a single patient and those mechanisms have interrelated effects. This section reviews

Table 1 Pediatric scoring system incorporating hepatic dysfunction in their model

Scoring system	Liver component	Cut-offs used in the prediction model
pSOFA [15]	Total bilirubin	Graded scale with increasing trend in mortality >20 μmol/L (1 point), >34 μmol/L (2 points), >103 μmol/L (3 points), >205 μmol/L (4 points)
P-MODS [16]	Total bilirubin	Graded scale with increasing trend in mortality >8.5 μmol (1 point), >34 μmol/L (2 points), >85.5 μmol/L (3 points), >171 μmol/L (4 points)
PRISM [17]	PT / PTT	PT > 22 s PTT > 57 s (85 s for neonates)

four major pathophysiological pathways of secondary liver injury in the critically ill children: hypoxic liver injury, sepsis and the systemic inflammatory response syndrome, venous congestion, and treatment-associated liver injury.

Hypoxic Liver Injury

Hypoxic liver injury occurs when oxygen supply to the liver fails to meet hepatic cells' demand. This type of liver injury is also named ischemic hepatitis, shock liver, or more recently hypoxic hepatitis. However, hypoxic liver injury is a broader term more representative of the multiple mechanisms that can lead to inadequate hepatocytes oxygen uptake.

In physiological conditions, the liver is relatively well protected from ischemia because of its dual blood perfusion: 75% of its blood flow is provided by the portal vein while the remaining 25% is provided by the hepatic artery. When cardiac blood flow decreases, the decreasing portal blood flow causes adenosine accumulation in the hepatic vasculature, which produces compensatory arteriolar dilation, a mechanism termed "hepatic arterial buffer response" (HABR) [18]. Additionally, the liver sinusoids are highly permeable and allow easier diffusion of oxygen to the hepatocytes, increasing their oxygen extraction capacity [18, 19]. These unique characteristics of the hepatic vasculature explain why a pure hypovolemic or hypoxic episode rarely causes hypoxic liver injury in otherwise healthy patients. However, in the intensive care population, patients often have underlying illnesses, so these compensatory mechanisms can be overwhelmed.

Fig. 1 Determinants of oxygen delivery

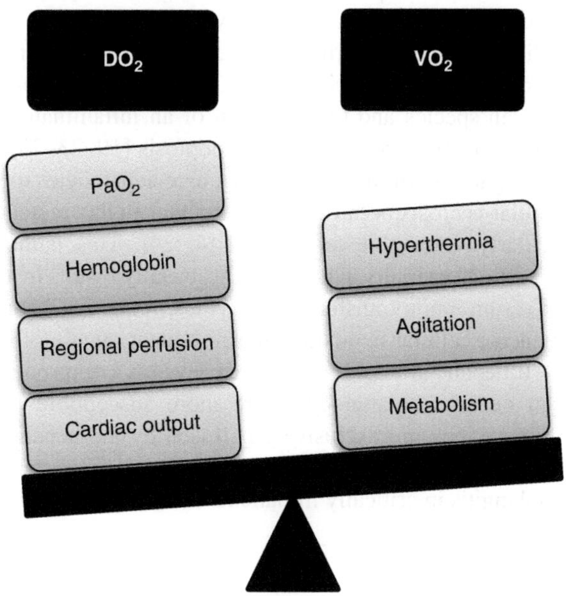

Insufficient oxygen supply to hepatocytes may be due to low systemic oxygen delivery (DO_2), increased oxygen consumption (VO_2), impaired oxygen use, or any combination of the above (Fig. 1).

Low cardiac output resulting in decreased hepatic blood flow is the most frequent cause of hypoxic liver injury and can occur in patients with heart failure or other types of shock. Indeed, the mesenteric circulation is distinctly affected by the systemic vasoconstriction produced by the neurohormonal activation in response to decreasing cardiac output [20]. The blood flow decrease must be severe enough to overcome the abovementioned compensation mechanisms. However, overt hypotension is documented in only 50% of adult patients with hypoxic hepatitis [5, 19]. This means that milder decrease in hepatic blood flow can lead to hypoxic injury if the liver is already vulnerable because of other causes of low DO_2 (severe hypoxemia, severe anemia), high VO_2 (hyperthermia), or impaired oxygen utilization (sepsis). Another common predisposing factor is the presence of passive hepatic congestion, which impairs oxygen diffusion by reducing sinusoidal perfusion pressure. This is frequently seen in patients with acute or acute on chronic heart failure with high central venous pressure and is further discussed below. Almost 75% of ICU patients with hypoxic liver injury have more than one underlying cause [21], reflecting the complex pathophysiological interactions in critically ill individuals. The presence of hypoxic liver injury in a normotensive patient can thus signal an "occult hypoperfusion" that must be addressed.

As stated above, reduction of hepatic blood flow is not the only mechanism that can cause hypoxic liver injury. Low DO_2 can also result from severe hypoxemia. In adult series, respiratory failure is found as the cause of hypoxic liver injury in 6–15% of patients, and very low levels of arterial pressure of oxygen are reported ($PaO_2 < 40$ mmHg) [6, 7, 19, 21, 22]. Patients with acute on chronic disease are especially at risk, probably because of the contribution of passive congestion if secondary right ventricular failure is present.

Besides the hepatic hypoperfusion per se, reperfusion injury is also an important mechanism of liver damage in hypoxic liver injury. Ischemia-reperfusion injury is defined as the exacerbation of cellular dysfunction following the restoration of blood flow after a period of lack of oxygen. It involves the generation of reactive oxygen species and the initiation of an inflammatory cascade leading to Kupffer cells activation, cell injury, and apoptosis [19, 23–25].

Regardless of the cause, inadequate hepatocytes oxygen uptake results in centrilobular necrosis because the hepatocytes in this metabolically active region are particularly vulnerable to hypoxia [4, 24]. This pathological pattern is typical of hypoxic liver injury. Clinically, this usually results in a severe but transient elevation of serum aminotransferases enzymes, reflecting hepatocellular necrosis provoked by acute cellular hypoxia with subsequent release of intracellular enzymes.

If hepatic arterial blood flow is severely compromised, ischemic cholangiopathy can occur. Cholangiocytes are more susceptible to ischemia than hepatocytes because they are exclusively perfused by the hepatic artery and are thus not protected by the hepatic dual blood perfusion. This can lead to secondary sclerosing cholangitis in critically ill patients (SCC-CIP), which is further discussed below.

Sepsis and Inflammation

The liver plays an important role in the systemic response to infection as a first line of defense against microorganisms entering from the gastrointestinal tract or from the systemic circulation. Indeed, Kupffer cells, which are resident macrophages lining the walls of the hepatic sinusoids, are favorably located to scavenge bacteria and endotoxins from the bloodstream. Kupffer cells are also able to recognize and respond to antigens, danger signals, and microorganisms products by the initiation of an immune response and the liberation of many acute phase mediators. While these mechanisms are crucial in host response to infection, dysregulated inflammation can in turn target the liver itself. Sepsis-induced liver injury is frequent (up to 1/3 of patients) and is known to be associated with poorer prognosis [26].

Sepsis and the systemic inflammatory response syndrome (SIRS) can lead to liver injury by many mechanisms (Fig. 2). As exposed above, any cause of shock can lead to hypoxic liver injury if oxygen supply to the liver fails to meet hepatic cells demand. Sepsis is a frequent cause of hypoxic hepatitis and is stated as the underlying cause in 6% to 33% of cases [25]. Typically, hepatosplanchnic blood flow is increased in sepsis because of decreased systemic vascular resistance. It is thus proposed that impaired oxygen extraction and utilization secondary to inflammation-induced mitochondrial dysfunction is the main mechanism of DO_2/VO_2 imbalance in this setting. However, sepsis can also impair oxygen delivery by secondary cardiac dysfunction, a common situation especially in the pediatric patient. Besides, the above-mentioned hepatic arterial buffer response (HABR) is compromised by endotoxin-induced endothelial dysfunction. Indeed, activated

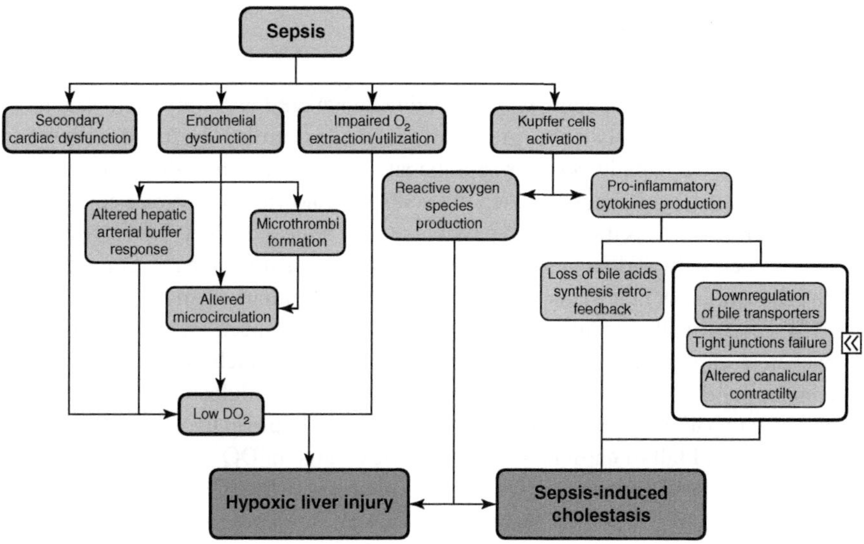

Fig. 2 Sepsis-induced liver injury

Kupffer cells and liver sinusoidal endothelial cells (LSEC) upregulate inducible NO synthase (iNOS), which impairs vasodilatory response and contributes to decreasing hepatic blood flow. Endothelial dysfunction, coupled with microthrombi formation, also leads to a severely impaired microcirculation that further enhances liver ischemia. As mentioned above, this type of liver injury usually presents as a "hepatocellular" type of liver test disturbance.

Another important mechanism of sepsis-associated liver dysfunction is a form of nonobstructive intrahepatic cholestasis. Cholestatic liver dysfunction is traditionally viewed as the most frequent type of liver injury in the setting of sepsis [26, 27]. Sepsis causes multiple disturbances in bile acids hepatobiliary transport and synthesis regulation. First, endotoxins like lipopolysaccharides (LPS) derived from Gram-negative bacteria or lipoprotein and teichoic acid derived from Gram-positive bacteria activate Kupffer cells. This triggers the production of multiple inflammatory cytokines (TNF-a, IL-1, IL-6, IL-12, IL-18), which leads to the downregulation of many important hepatobiliary transporters [11, 27–30]. The resulting impairment in bile flow is further enhanced by an iNOs-mediated increase in the permeability of hepatocytes tight junctions. This alters the hepatocyte's cell polarity and thus compromises bile excretion. Canalicular contraction is also affected, leading to biliary sludge and slower bile transport. Inflammation also causes loss of retro-feedback mechanisms on bile acid synthesis, increasing bile acid overload.

Finally, Kupffer cells activation and pro-inflammatory cytokines can produce ongoing parenchymal and endothelial injury from the release of reactive oxygen species and proteases. This can aggravate both hepatocellular injury and cholestasis.

Venous Congestion

Passive liver congestion occurs when hepatic venous outflow is impaired. The most common cause for this is right-sided or biventricular cardiac dysfunction, but any obstruction of the hepatic veins or suprahepatic vena cava could also result in congestive hepatopathy. Because the hepatic veins have no valves, central venous pressure (CVP) elevation is transmitted passively to the sinusoidal bed. This predisposes to liver ischemia by reducing sinusoidal perfusion pressure and by causing dilation of the sinusoids, which leads to stasis and microthrombus formation [5, 11, 19, 31–33]. Usually, this could be compensated by enhanced oxygen extraction. However, if cardiac anterograde flow is compromised, which is often the case in decompensated heart failure, liver hypoxia, and hepatocellular injury ensue. This explains why patients with elevated CVP can develop hypoxic liver injury even with a relatively mild fall of cardiac output or subtle change in DO_2.

Many adult studies support the central role of elevated CVP in hypoxic liver injury. Hemodynamic studies have shown that elevated central filling pressure is present in the majority of patients with hypoxic liver injury [22, 34, 35]. Cardiac failure is also the most frequently identified underlying cause of hypoxic hepatitis in this population, with prevalence ranging from 39–70% [19, 22, 23, 35]. In children, it is often seen following cardiac surgery, especially in patients with right-sided pathology like Tetralogy of Fallot [10]. The role of venous congestion in the pathophysiology of hypoxic liver injury can explain why it is often observed in cardiogenic shock but rarely in pure hypovolemic or hemorrhagic shock.

Prolonged elevation of central venous pressure can also cause a congestive hepatopathy, as seen in patients with chronic right-sided heart failure, certain congenital heart malformations, functional single ventricule, and Fontan palliation. In these cases, the chronic dilation of the sinusoids stimulates the stellate cells to produce a fibrotic reaction, and the chronic stasis promotes thrombi formation leading to hypoxia and liver fibrosis [32]. Hepatocytes chronically compensate with an increased oxygen extraction rate, but are thus very vulnerable to any supplemental insults. In this setting, even a minor deterioration of cardiac function and forward flow could lead to severe and acute hepatocellular injury. Heart-liver interactions are further discussed in the Chapter Liver failure and the heart.

Treatment-Associated Liver Injury

Patients often require multiple treatments and pharmacological agents over the course of their ICU stay. Many of these treatments can contribute to the development or aggravation of liver injury. Of those, parenteral nutrition-associated liver disease (PNLAD), drug-induced liver injury (DILI) and liver injury associated with transfusion are of particular interest and will be discussed below.

Parenteral Nutrition-Associated Liver Disease (PNLAD)

Parenteral nutrition (PN) is often needed in critically ill children when enteral feeding is either contraindicated, not tolerated, or insufficient to provide adequate nutrient and caloric intake. While this nutritional support is essential and sometimes lifesaving, one of its main adverse effect is the development of liver injury, specifically cholestasis. The incidence of PNLAD in children is around 30% [36]. The development of PNLAD is closely related to the duration of PN: it occurs in 15% of patients receiving PN for 14–30 days but in up to 60% of patients receiving PN for >60 days [36]. Other important risks factors include prematurity/low birth weight, an underlying surgical condition (necrotizing enterocolitis, gastroschisis, intestinal atresia), sepsis, higher daily total caloric intake, higher lipid content, and the absence of any enteral feeding [37, 38]. Children typically develop PNLAD faster than adults, probably because of already immature hepatobiliary and intestinal function and because of higher energy requirements [39].

The pathophysiology of PNLAD is not fully understood and is clearly a complex multifactorial phenomenon. Central to its development is the impact of absence of enteral feeding, which causes multiple physiological impairments. First, it profoundly alters the gut microbiota and favors the growth of pathogenic bacteria, which stimulates pro-inflammatory cytokines and compromises the intestinal epithelium integrity [39]. Mucosal atrophy from the absence of luminal nutriments further jeopardizes the epithelial barrier function. Intestinal motility is also decreased, which encourages intraluminal bacterial overgrowth. Combined with increased intestinal permeability, this promotes bacterial and endotoxin translocation to the portal circulation and liver inflammation, causing liver injury directly, but also through cytokine-mediated alteration in bile production and transport [40]. The absence of enteral nutrition also alters specific signaling between the gut and the liver which contributes to bile transport anomalies. Multiple studies show that PNLAD can be minimized by preservation of at least trophic feedings. Progression of enteral feeding is the best treatment of PNLAD. There is also some data suggesting that cyclic parental nutrition (providing an off-time of 1 to 2-h each day) is effective in the prevention and treatment of this condition [37, 41].

PN itself is associated with an increased production of pro-inflammatory cytokines. This has been mainly attributed to the use of intravenous lipid emulsions, especially those that are rich in omega-6 polyunsaturated fatty acids because of their pro-inflammatory derivatives. Phytosterols contained in those fat emulsions are also a factor in the development of PNLAD. Some strategies to minimize this type of liver damage include lipid restriction and the use of alternative lipid emulsions like fish oil-based lipid emulsions (Omegaven®) or SMOF lipids [42, 43]. There is a need for more data on the effectiveness of those strategies in children outside of the neonatal period.

PNLAD typically manifests as different degrees of cholestasis with elevation of conjugated bilirubin, alkaline phosphatase, and gamma-glutamyl transferase. A mixed pattern with cholestasis and transaminases elevation is also possible. Histologically, intrahepatic cholestasis and liver steatosis are the characteristic findings. Those anomalies are usually benign and reversible following discontinuation of PN and resumption of feeding, except in very severe cases (e.g. intestinal-failure associated end-stage liver disease).

Drug-Induced Liver Injury (DILI)

DILI is a frequent cause of liver injury in the general population: it represents 10–25% of acute hepatitis and is the most common cause of acute liver failure in developed countries [4, 44]. It accounts for almost 20% of pediatric acute liver failure [45]. Being the primary site of drug metabolism, the liver is especially susceptible to drug-induced injury. Hepatic metabolism of drugs and xenobiotics follows three principal steps: First, in phase 1 reactions, drugs are transformed to active and possibly toxic metabolites. In phase 2, reactions neutralize those metabolites by conjugation pathways, enabling the phase 3, i.e. their secretion and elimination. Accumulation of phase 1 metabolites can lead to DILI [45]. The two main categories of DILI are direct or intrinsic hepatotoxicity and idiosyncratic drug reactions. In intrinsic hepatotoxicity, the drug or its metabolite causes hepatocellular necrosis in a predictable and dose-dependent fashion. On the contrary, idiosyncratic reactions, which are responsible for the majority of DILI cases, are unpredictable, dose independent, and have very variable latency. Those type of reactions result from immune (hypersensibility reactions) or nonimmune mechanism (genetically determined variation in drug metabolism), or a combination of both.

DILI can lead to hepatocellular, cholestatic, or a mixed pattern of liver injury. In the DILIN Prospective Study [46], a longitudinal multicenter study exploring DILI in children, the pattern of injury was hepatocellular in 78% of DILI episodes. The clinical picture can range from asymptomatic liver test anomalies to acute liver failure [47]. It can be difficult to distinguish from other causes of liver injury and remains a diagnostic of exclusion. Symptoms vary depending on the severity and pattern of injury. If the cause of DILI is an immune mechanism, symptoms related to hypersensibility reactions may appear, like fever, rash, and arthralgia. An improvement of liver test after discontinuation of the culprit drug is an important clue to diagnosis, but the time to recovery is variable, ranging from days to months [45, 46].

Critically ill patients are particularly vulnerable to DILI for many reasons. First, these patients are exposed to a high number of drugs and agents, which can lead to drug interactions but also multiplies potential toxic effects. Second, the systemic inflammatory state seen in critical illness can alter hepatic drug metabolism and lead to a reduction of important detoxification and elimination reactions (phase 2 reactions), thus increasing the toxic effect of some metabolites [11]. Finally, as discussed above, patients admitted to the ICU are subject to many other forms of hepatic insults (hypoxic liver injury, inflammation, congestion) that sensitizes hepatic cell to injury.

A multitude of drugs can lead to DILI. Table 2 summarizes drugs that are commonly used in the pediatric ICU that can cause liver injury. Many resources provide details on drug-induced hepatotoxicity, including LiverTox [48], an internet database that contains information of prescription and over-the-counter drugs implicated in DILI. In the DILIN pediatric cohort [46], antimicrobial was the most commonly implicated drug class (50% of DILI episodes), followed shortly by CNS agents (40% of episodes).

Transfusions

There is emerging data regarding the possibility of a so-called transfusion-related acute hepatic injury or TRAHI. A pediatric study found a relationship between platelets transfusion in patients post Fontan surgery and acute hepatic injury [50]. Another small adult study [51] found that an elevation of liver enzymes after blood transfusion was common. The pathophysiology could be similar to TRALI

Table 2 Common medications used in the PICU that can cause liver injury

Drug	Mechanism	Pattern	LiverTox category[a]	Particularities
Antimicrobials				
Minocycline	Idiosyncratic	Hepatocellular	A	Most common implicated drug in DILIN study (13% of episodes) Possible auto-immune hepatitis-like presentation
Ketoconazole	Idiosyncratic	Hepatocellular	A	
Isoniazid	Idiosyncratic	Hepatocellular	A	Surveillance monitoring is controversial
Macrolides	Idiosyncratic	Cholestasis	A	
Amoxicillin/clavulanate	Idiosyncratic	Cholestasis	A	Most common cause of DILI worldwide
Trimethoprim-sulfamethoxazole	Idiosyncratic	Mixed	Not classified	
Clindamycine	Idiosyncratic Direct	Mixed	B	Mild direct injury during high dose IV therapy Idiosyncratic reaction similar to other antibiotics
Rifampin	Idiosyncratic	Hepatocellular	A	
Antiepileptics				
Phenytoin	Idiosyncratic	Mixed	A	Can occur in the context of a drug rash with eosinophilia and systemic symptoms (DRESS)
Valproic acid	Idiosyncratic (mitochondrial toxicity?)	Hepatocellular	A	Children <2 years old are more vulnerable Possible role of L-carnitine for treatment
Carbamazepine	Idiosyncratic	Mixed	A	
Phenobarbital	Idiosyncratic	Mixed	B	
Others				
Acetaminophen	Direct	Hepatocellular	A	Most common drug causing acute DILI in America Specific treatment protocols (N acetyl cysteine)
Amiodarone	Idiosyncratic	Hepatocellular	A	Surveillance monitoring is recommended

Table 2 (continued)

Drug	Mechanism	Pattern	LiverTox category[a]	Particularities
Propofol	Idiosyncratic	Hepatocellular	Not classified	Overlap with propofol infusion syndrome
Methotrexate	Idiosyncratic	Hepatocellular	A	Surveillance monitoring is recommended

Adapted from Horvatitis et al. [4], Amin et al. [45], Molleston et al. [46] and Lescot et al. [49]
[a]LiverTox categories [48]; Category A: well known to cause liver injury, Category B: known or highly likely to cause liver injury

(transfusion-related acute lung injury), with blood products causing neutrophils and endothelium activation and increased vascular permeability.

Clinical Presentation and Patterns of Acquired Liver Injury and Failure

Patterns of Liver Injury

While there are multiple causes of hepatic dysfunction in critical care, most patients will display one of three patterns: hepatocellular injury, cholestatic dysfunction, or less frequently secondary sclerosing cholangitis (SSC-CIP). The characteristics of those three patterns of injury are summarized in Table 3. *Hepatocellular injury* is characterized by injury to the hepatocytes and causes a rapid elevation of serum aminotransferases enzymes (AST and ALT). Clinically, it can present as asymptomatic laboratory anomalies, acute hepatic synthetic dysfunction or even acute liver failure (ALF). *Cholestatic injury* is characterized by an alteration of bile clearance and causes accumulation of bile acids, conjugated bilirubin, and alkaline phosphatase (ALP) in the blood. Depending on the severity, it can be asymptomatic or can lead to the clinical picture of jaundice. *Secondary sclerosing* cholangitis in critically ill patients (SSC-CIP) is a rare but severe form of liver injury where cholangiocytes injury leads to progressive biliary damage and sclerosing cholangitis. Two principal mechanisms lead to cholangiocytes injury: severe ischemia (described above in the hypoxic hepatitis section) and toxicity from biliary components during cholestasis and systemic inflammation. This leads to cholangiocyte necrosis and progressive obstruction of the intrahepatic bile ducts, eventually leading to biliary cirrhosis [52]. Patients with SCC-CIP are typically survivors of severe critical illness who needed mechanical ventilation and hemodynamic support. The clinical presentation is persistent cholestasis beyond the period that is expected for cholestatic injury and a rapid progression to cirrhosis and liver failure with a high mortality rate [4, 11, 53].

Table 3 Patterns of liver injury in the ICU

	Hepatocellular	Cholestatic	SSC-CIP
Physiopathology and pattern	Hepatocytes injury +/− necrosis Acute elevation of AST/ALT	Alteration of bile synthesis, secretion of excretion Elevation of conjugated bilirubin, GGT, and ALP	Cholangiocytes necrosis Obliteration of intrahepatic bile ducts
Main causes in the ICU	Hypoxic liver injury Congestive hepatopathy Sepsis Drugs (DILI)	Sepsis Parental nutrition Drugs (DILI)	Severe hemodynamic instability
Clinical presentation	Asymptomatic Synthetic dysfunction Acute hepatic failure (ALF)	Asymptomatic Elimination dysfunction Acalculous cholecystitis Acute hepatic failure (rare)	Persistent cholestasis Progressive cirrhosis Chronic liver failure High risk of cholangitis
Timing	Early and acute Peak 24–48 h after insult Slow decrease over 10 days	Subacute Days into ICU stay	Persistent after episode of instability Progressive cirrhosis over weeks/months

Clinical Presentation and Evolution

The clinical presentation of acquired liver injury in critically ill patients can range from asymptomatic laboratory anomalies to full-blown acute liver failure with encephalopathy. Secondary sclerosing cholangitis exhibit a specific clinical presentation and is discussed above.

Acute liver failure (ALF) can occur in up to 25% of adult patients with hypoxic liver injury but is rare in the other pathophysiological mechanisms [4]. The diagnosis of ALF in patients with hypoxic liver injury is difficult since many of these patients have some degree of encephalopathy because of their underlying illness, and a lot of them are sedated. The INR criteria is also difficult to interpret in patients with shock or sepsis-associated disseminated intravascular coagulation. Hyperammonemia seems to be relatively frequent in patients with hypoxic liver injury, but rarely causes cerebral edema [23, 24].

Even when the clinical severity does not reach ALF criteria, acute liver dysfunction can have multiple clinical consequences in critically ill patients. First, the metabolism and excretion of drugs can be altered, which can increase the risk of drug toxicity and drug-induced liver injury. Liver dysfunction can also cause or worsen coagulation and bleeding disorders and leads to an altered immune response and an increased incidence of infections [54]. Children are particularly prone to the development of hypoglycemia, which can occur in up to 50% of patients in this context and needs to be closely monitored [19].

ICU patients with acquired liver injury, especially hypoxic liver injury, can present with impaired oxygenation because of the hepatopulmonary syndrome. While this syndrome is well-recognized in cirrhotic patients, it can also occur in acute liver injury and was found in 46% of ICU patients with hypoxic liver injury in an adult study [55]. The hepatopulmonary syndrome consists of intrapulmonary vascular vasodilation and pulmonary arteriovenous communications with right-to-left shunting which aggravates hypoxemia in patients often already requiring respiratory support. This seems to be entirely reversible when normalization of hepatic function occurs if the underlying disease is treated [4, 55].

Acute kidney injury occurs in up to 80% of ICU patients with hypoxic liver injury. Many of those patients will need renal replacement therapy. Kidney injury in patients with acute liver failure or dysfunction is usually multifactorial and frequently reversible following normalization of hepatic function and treatment of the underlying disorder. The development of kidney injury in patients with hypoxic liver injury is an independent predictor of mortality in adults [56].

Finally, cholestasis increases the risk of acalculous cholecystitis. ICU patients are already vulnerable to this disease because of fasting, total parenteral nutrition, ischemia, and SIRS. Gallbladder stasis leads to concentration of irritating bile salts and to its distension, with following necrosis and risk of perforation. Clinically, this can present as classic symptoms of acute cholecystitis (right upper quadrant pain, Murphy's sign, nausea, vomiting, food intolerance), fever, or signs of sepsis and shock.

Diagnosis

Hypoxic Liver Injury

The diagnosis of hypoxic liver injury is based on the presence of three criteria [19, 23–25]

1. A clinical setting prone to causing inadequate oxygen uptake by the hepatocytes (acute cardiac, circulatory or respiratory failure).
2. An acute and massive rise in serum aminotransferase. Most authors used a cut-off of >20 times the upper limit of normal.
3. Exclusion of other causes of acute liver necrosis (for example acute-on-chronic liver failure, viral hepatitis, drug-induced liver injury).

When patients meet these criteria, it is widely accepted that liver biopsy is usually not warranted. Some studies have proposed lower cut-off values of aminotransferase such as 5 or 10 times the upper limit of normal [5, 6, 22, 49]. Other authors maintain that a histologic confirmation should be obtained when those lower cut-off values are used, but there is no consensus. Performing a liver biopsy in critically ill patients can be problematic, especially if there is a significant coagulopathy, and is thus often reserved to atypical cases. If it is done, the classical pattern is centrilobular liver cell necrosis, particularly involving the area around the central vein (zone III), without the presence of inflammatory cells [11, 23, 24]. Features of passive congestion like sinusoids dilation can also be observed.

Patients with hypoxic liver injury usually display a typical pattern of laboratory findings that can help to differentiate this type of liver injury from other causes like DILI or viral hepatitis. First, there is a dramatic rise of transaminase early after the precipitating event (8–24 h). This rise usually peaks in the first 48–72 h, with aspartate aminotransferase (AST) levels initially higher than alanine aminotransferase (ALT). Approximately 75% of ICU patients with hypoxic liver injury present the above-mentioned diagnostic criteria on the first day of admission [12, 21, 57], which highlights the rapidity of hypoxic hepatitis after the original insult. Another distinctive feature of hypoxic liver injury is the early and marked rise in lactate dehydrogenase (LDH). It has been proposed that an ALT-to-LDH ratio less than 1.5 could distinguish hypoxic liver injury from viral or drug-induced hepatitis [11, 24]. The increase in the international normalized ratio (INR) usually occurs after the transaminase peak. Perturbation in INR is usually of lesser amplitude than the perturbation in aminotransferases levels but can reach levels defining acute liver failure in severe cases. Once the underlying cause is corrected, AST and ALT rapidly fall (often by >50% within 72 h) and gradually normalize in 7–10 days. AST levels tend to normalize faster because their half-life (17 h) is shorter than ALT (50 h) [23, 24, 49]. Thirty percent of the patients develop clinical jaundice after the initial rise in ALT/AST [57].

Abdominal ultrasound can be useful in demonstrating features of venous congestion, like dilation of the inferior vena cava and of the suprahepatic veins. Patients in which a diagnosis of hypoxic liver injury is made should also undergo echocardiography to assess cardiac function and, depending on the clinical setting and the severity of illness, invasive hemodynamic assessment should be considered [11, 23].

Cholestatic Liver Dysfunction

The criteria for the diagnosis of cholestatic liver dysfunction in critically ill patients are less defined. Most studies use a total bilirubin higher than 34 μmol/L (>2 mg/dL) [2, 4, 30, 58], which is derived from studies in adults and in children with cirrhosis. However, the only pediatric study on critical illness-induced cholestasis demonstrated an increase in mortality starting at bilirubin level as low as 13 μmol/L[9], questioning the transferability of the adult definition to children. Further studies are needed to confirm this potential difference in the pediatric population. Alkaline phosphatase (ALP) and gamma glutamyl transpeptidase (GGT) are two other commonly used and sensitive indicators of cholestasis. Values >2–3 times the upper limit of normal are usually considered for the diagnosis [4, 30, 49].

All patients with cholestatic liver dysfunction should have an abdominal ultrasound to rule out biliary obstruction. If there is a persistent cholestasis beyond recovery from the acute illness, secondary sclerosing cholangiopathy (SSC) must be considered and additional imaging must be performed. Magnetic resonance cholangiopancreatography (MRCP) is a good exam and can show biliary casts and strictures. The gold standard for the diagnosis of SSC-CIP remains endoscopic retrograde cholangiopancreatography (ERCP).

Pitfalls in Diagnosis

One of the main challenges in the diagnosis of liver injury in critically ill patients is the lack of specificity of the common liver laboratory tests. This is especially true for complex ICU patients who have many physiologic perturbations and treatment that could impact those lab results.

Aminotransferases

Aspartate aminotransferase (AST) and alanine aminotransferase (ALT) are intracellular enzymes that are released into plasma upon liver injury and their elevation suggests hepatocellular injury or necrosis. However, AST is not specific to the liver and is present is many other organs like the heart, muscles, kidney, pancreas, erythrocytes, and leukocytes. In ICU patients, elevated AST can be due to many nonhepatic alterations, for example, poor tissue perfusion, myopathy, and cardiac ischemia. ALT is more specific to the liver and its elevation suggests hepatocellular injury. However, the magnitude of aminotransferase elevation correlates poorly with the severity of liver necrosis or, even more importantly, with the severity of hepatic dysfunction.

Bilirubin

Serum bilirubin is frequently used as a marker of cholestasis and as an indicator of hepatic excretory function. However, elevated serum bilirubin can be due to multiple processes: (1) increased production (hemolysis, transfusions); (2) impaired uptake, conjugation, and or/excretion by the liver (hepatic dysfunction); or (3) posthepatic obstruction (intra- or extra-hepatic biliary obstruction) [57, 59]. The measurement of the direct portion or conjugated bilirubin can help to differentiate pre-hepatic from intra- or post-hepatic obstruction, as it reflects primarily the excretion function and indicate a preservation of the conjugation function. Serum bilirubin is the most common liver test to be included in scoring algorithms and is known to correlate with ICU outcome [1, 2, 58]. However, it is a late marker of hepatic dysfunction and lacks sensitivity to detect less-severe hepatic injury [11, 49, 57].

Alkaline Phosphatase

Alkaline phosphatase (ALP) is an intracellular enzyme derived mainly from hepatocytes, cholangiocytes, and bone. Retained biliary acids during cholestasis stimulate production of ALP and its release in the circulation. As levels are physiologically higher in childhood, it is important to use specific pediatric reference values. ALP is very sensitive for cholestasis, but has low specificity and can also be elevated in high bone turnover conditions (for example fractures, rickets, osteomyelitis, hyperthyroidism). If there is an isolated elevation in ALP, measurement of gamma-glutamyltransferase (GGT) can help to differentiate a hepatic from a bony origin [59]. Indeed, GGT is not specific to the liver as it is also found in the kidney, intestine, prostate, and pancreas, but it is not found in bone. Similar to ALP, GGT is very sensitive to cholestasis.

INR

The prothrombin time (expressed as the INR) measures the activity of the coagulation factors of the intrinsic pathway, including factor II, V, VII, X. As all these factors are produced by the liver, the INR can reflect the hepatic synthetic capacity. However, in the ICU setting, an elevated INR can be caused by many other factors like disseminated intravascular coagulation, massive bleeding, vitamin K deficiency, and hemodilution [49].

Albumin

Because it is synthetized only by the hepatocytes, albumin can also be used to reflect the liver's synthetic function. However, it is not useful in critically ill patients because albumin serum concentration is dependent on too many confounding factors: albumin production (malnutrition, acute phase response), compartment shifts and distribution (hemodilution, increased vascular permeability, blood loss), or increased catabolism in stress states. [11, 49, 57, 59] Thus, it should not be used as a specific test of hepatic function in this population.

Novel Markers and Tests

To overcome diagnostic problems related to the lack of specificity of classic liver blood tests, research is ongoing to find novel markers of hepatic dysfunction. There is a need to find tests that can better assess the extent of liver dysfunction at the bedside and are less prone to the numerous confounding factors in the ICU context.

Serum Bile Acids Levels

Bile acids are produced in the liver from cholesterol, and are secreted in the intestine in their primary form with bile where they are converted to secondary bile acids by the action of the gut bacterial flora. They are then re-absorbed in ileum and transported back to the liver (the entero-hepatic circulation). As explained in the pathophysiology section, the main mechanism of critical illness-induced cholestasis seems to be related to multiple disturbances in bile acids hepatobiliary transport, synthesis regulation, and retro feedback. It is thus believed that serum bile acids levels could indicate the presence of cholestasis earlier and more specifically than bilirubin [4, 30, 57]. In a study of critically ill adults, total bile acids levels predicted short-term mortality better than bilirubin levels [60]. Serum total bile acids level is available in most labs and is already used in the diagnosis of intrahepatic cholestasis of pregnancy [61]. The serum bile acids profile (individual levels or primary and secondary bile acids) could provide additional information but is not currently available in clinical practice. More data is needed on the signification of individual bile acids levels in critically ill patients.

Indocyanine Green Plasma Disappearance Rate (ICG-PDR)

Indocyanine green is a nontoxic water-soluble tricarbocyanine dye that is eliminated exclusively by the liver and secreted into bile unchanged without enterohepatic circulation. Its elimination rate thus reflects the elimination function of the liver, and the ICG-PDR has been developed to be used as a dynamic test of liver function. It was described as early as 1960, but the recent development of a noninvasive technique using transcutaneous spectrophotometry with results available within a few minutes at the bedside has renewed interest for its clinical use [25, 49, 62]. The results are expressed as percentage of concentration change over time, with the initial concentration being 100%. Normal values above 18%/min have been reported [63]. ICG-PDR can be used to assess liver function post hepatic resection and post liver transplant. In the past years, an ICG-PDR <8%/min was found to be a good and independent prognostic marker of survival in critically ill patients [62, 64–66]. Its sensitivity and specificity in predicting mortality seems to be similar to complex scoring systems like the APACHE score [66] and superior to standard biochemical tests like transaminases and bilirubin [65]. Specifically in critically ill patients with hypoxic hepatitis, there is a strong association between ICG-PDR and 28-day mortality. At 48 h after admission, ICG-PDR was superior to the SOFA score and to standard tests of liver function like INR in predicting mortality. Survivors displayed a constant increase in ICG clearance over time, while nonsurvivors failed to show this improvement [67]. One limitation of this test is that indocyanine green's excretion depends not only on the hepatic function but also on the hepatic blood flow, and some authors have questioned its value in situations of altered hepatic flow [57, 68]. Further studies are needed to better explore this limitation and the clinical role of ICG-PDR in liver function analysis.

Liver Stiffness

The evaluation of liver stiffness by transient elastography is a technique that is mostly used for the evaluation of hepatic fibrosis in patients with chronic liver disease as a noninvasive alternative to liver biopsy. Liver stiffness is also significantly increased in critically ill noncirrhotic patients and can reach levels usually seen in advanced hepatic disease. Values >18 kPa at ICU admission are associated with increased mortality and could be useful to detect early hepatic dysfunction [69]. However, the measurement could not be adequately performed in up to 30% of ICU patients, and some confounders exists (edema and fluid overload). Additional studies are needed to better appreciate the application of this technique to critically ill patients.

An Approach to Abnormal Liver Tests in the ICU

When faced with abnormal liver tests in a critically ill child, the first step, if not already done, is to repeat a complete panel of standard liver test, including AST, ALT, GGT, ALP, total and conjugated bilirubin, albumin, and a coagulation panel. The clinician can then define the predominant pattern of liver injury: hepatocellular injury (mainly elevated ALT/AST) or cholestatic injury (elevated total and conjugated bilirubin, elevated ALP and GGT).

Figures 3 and 4 show a suggested diagnostic approach for hepatocellular and cholestatic injury in the critically ill patient. Importantly, this does not include the approach of cholestasis in the neonatal period, as the differential diagnosis in this period is quite different and include among other diagnosis inborn errors of metabolism, congenital biliary anomalies like biliary atresia and genetic intrahepatic cholestasis syndromes. Special consideration for these diagnoses is warranted for infants <6 months, especially if the cholestasis is present at admission and no previous hepatic tests are available. In case of doubt, consultation with a specialist in pediatric hepatology is suggested.

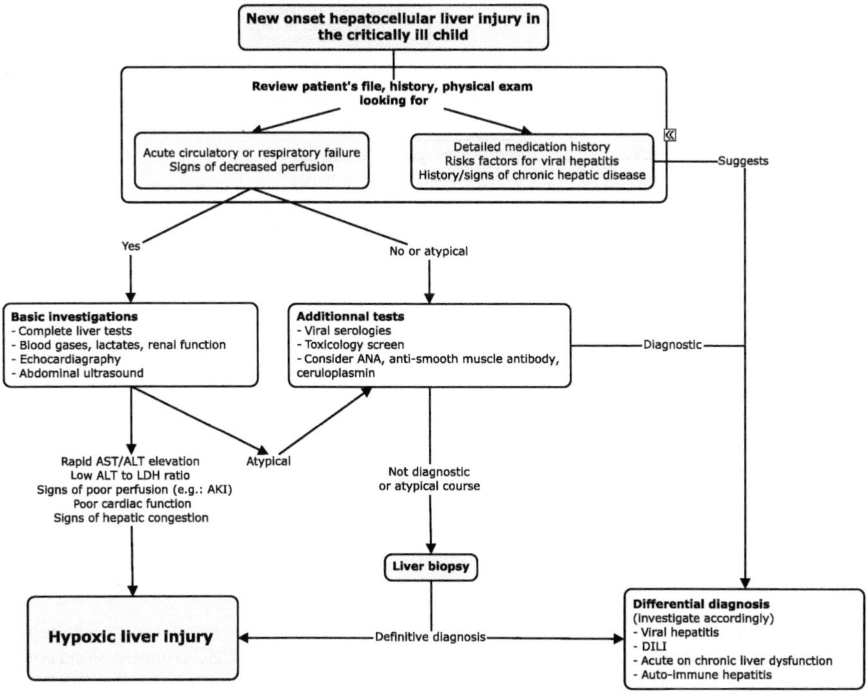

Fig. 3 Approach to hepatocellular injury in the critically ill child. ANA anti-nuclear antibodies, AKI acute kidney injury, DILI drug induced liver injury

Treatment

Treating the Underlying Cause and Preventing Further Injury

The most important component of the treatment of critical illness-induced liver injury is early recognition of abnormal liver tests and prompt identification and stabilization of the underlying illness. In hypoxic liver injury, the duration of increasing aminotransferase is strongly associated with outcome: patients in which the AST levels continue to increase after 24 h have higher mortality rates [21], emphasizing the importance of early recognition and treatment. Moreover, mild cholestasis can sometimes go unnoticed for many days in ICU patients with many abnormal laboratory tests, preventing early intervention. It is important that clinicians specifically look for cholestasis in critically ill patients and investigate patients accordingly.

Central to the treatment of ICU-acquired liver injury is the treatment of the underlying disease. This includes hemodynamic stabilization with an emphasis on optimization of liver perfusion and oxygen delivery. One of the challenges of hemodynamic resuscitation in this context is the preservation of the hepatosplanchnic circulation. Indeed, the use of vasopressors to optimize arterial pressure can worsen

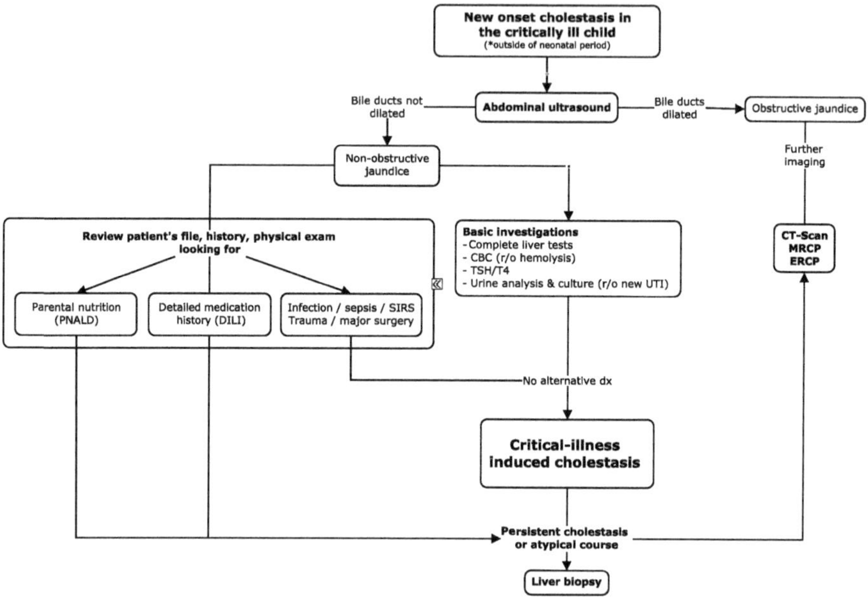

Fig. 4 Approach to cholestasis in the critically ill child. MRCP magnetic resonance cholangiopancreatography, ERCP endoscopic retrograde cholangiopancreatography, CBC compete blood count, PNALD Parenteral nutrition-associated liver disease, DILI drug-induced liver injury, SIRS systemic inflammatory response syndrome, dx diagnosis

the neurohormonally induced mesenteric vasoconstriction, further compromising hepatic arterial blood flow. While some potentially beneficial effects of dopamine and dobutamine [70, 71] have been suggested, no "ideal vasopressor" have been identified for patients with liver injury. Another important point is to avoid fluid overload, as hepatic congestion and high intra-abdominal pressure are two key mechanisms in the development of hypoxic liver injury. Any infection or sepsis should be aggressively treated with antimicrobial therapy and prompt source control.

To prevent further liver injury, the hepatosplanchnic blood flow should be preserved but how to achieve this goal remains a challenge and needs further research.

Additionally, a particular focus should be given to prevent further hepatic injury. A comprehensive review of the patient's medication list should be undertaken and potentially hepatotoxic drugs should be discontinued or replaced if clinically feasible. If the patient is on parenteral nutrition, some strategies can mitigate the associated cholestasis. The most effective strategy is enteral feeding and discontinuation of parenteral nutrition, but when full enteral feeding is not possible, even trophic feeding can improve PNALD. Other strategies can include lipid restriction to 1 g/kg/day, avoiding overcaloric parenteral nutrition, cycling of parenteral nutrition, and the use of alternative non-soybean-based lipid intravenous emulsions (ex: Omegaven®, SMOF lipids) [37]. Ursodeoxycholic acid is a hydrophilic bile acid that stimulates bile flow, reduces bile acid saturation, and decreases the cytotoxicity of hydrophobic acids. Administered orally, it has shown some positive effects for the prevention and treatment of PNLAD [36, 37, 42, 72], but data are scarce and further studies are needed on its efficacy.

Treating the Complications

Patients who develop consequences of liver dysfunction or failure are mostly treated with supportive measures. Glucose monitoring and glycemic control are crucial in critically ill children with liver injury. Both spontaneous hypoglycemia and hyperglycemia can occur and lead to deleterious consequences. Sustained hyperglycemia contributes to gallbladder dysmotility and one study showed a reduction of cholestasis and biliary sludge in critically ill patients in whom tight glycemic control by insulin therapy was instituted [3]. The optimal target for glycemic control in ICU patients is still up for debate, but in light of this data, a particular effort to avoid severe or sustained hyperglycemia should be undertaken in patients with cholestatic dysfunction.

Because of high incidence of acute kidney injury in patients with hypoxic liver injury, renal replacement therapies are frequently needed in this population [4, 73]. Advance dialysis devices like extracorporeal albumin dialysis with Molecular Absorbent Recirculating System technique (MARS) or Advanced Organ Support system (ADVOS) can be considered, but there is very little data on their use specifically in patients with hypoxic liver injury and further prospective studies are needed [74, 75]. For further details, see chapter on acute liver failure. However, there is a general consensus that acute liver failure caused by hypoxic liver injury is not an indication for liver transplant [76].

Specific Treatment and Research

Research is ongoing to find liver-specific therapy or prevention strategies for critical care-acquired liver injury, but strong clinical evidence is lacking at the moment. Ursodeoxycholic acid has been suggested for the treatment of sepsis-associated cholestasis and improved laboratory abnormalities [77, 78], but very few data are available for patients without PNLAD. Experimental data suggest that statins could improve liver microcirculation and prevent reperfusion injury, and one adult study showed that treatment with statin prior to ICU admission was a protective factor against hypoxic liver injury [4, 56]. Finally, N-acetylcysteine (NAC) seems to have clinical benefits in patients with non-acetaminophen acute liver failure [79, 80], but convincing evidence in hypoxic liver injury is lacking.

Conclusion

Liver injury and dysfunction is frequent in the pediatric intensive care unit and is associated with poorer outcomes. Multiple factors contribute to its development and often coexists in ICU patients, including hypoxic liver injury, venous congestion, sepsis, parenteral nutrition, and drug-induced liver injury. The diagnosis of acquired liver injury is a challenge in ICU patients because of multiple confounders and nonspecific markers. However, clinicians should specifically look for abnormal liver tests as early recognition and treatment of the underlying cause are key.

References

1. Thomson SJ, Cowan ML, Johnston I, Musa S, Grounds M, Rahman TM. 'Liver function tests' on the intensive care unit: a prospective, observational study. Intensive Care Med. 2009;35(8):1406–11. https://doi.org/10.1007/s00134-009-1511-7.
2. Kramer L, Jordan B, Druml W, Bauer P, Metnitz PGH, for the Austrian Epidemiologic Study on Intensive Care ASG. Incidence and prognosis of early hepatic dysfunction in critically ill patients—A prospective multicenter study. Crit Care Med. 2007;35(4):1099. https://doi.org/10.1097/01.CCM.0000259462.97164.A0.
3. Mesotten D, Wauters J, Van den Berghe G, Wouters PJ, Milants I, Wilmer A. The effect of strict blood glucose control on biliary sludge and cholestasis in critically ill patients. J Clin Endocrinol Metab. 2009;94(7):2345–52. https://doi.org/10.1210/jc.2008-2579.
4. Horvatits T, Drolz A, Trauner M, Fuhrmann V. Liver injury and failure in critical illness. Hepatology. 2019;70(6):2204–15. https://doi.org/10.1002/hep.30824.
5. Tapper EB, Sengupta N, Bonder A. The incidence and outcomes of ischemic hepatitis: a systematic review with meta-analysis. Am J Med. 2015;128(12):1314–21. https://doi.org/10.1016/j.amjmed.2015.07.033.
6. Van den Broecke A, Van Coile L, Decruyenaere A, et al. Epidemiology, causes, evolution and outcome in a single-center cohort of 1116 critically ill patients with hypoxic hepatitis. Ann Intensive Care. 2018;8:15. https://doi.org/10.1186/s13613-018-0356-z.
7. Aboelsoud MM, Javaid AI, Al-Qadi MO, Lewis JH. Hypoxic hepatitis — its biochemical profile, causes and risk factors of mortality in critically-ill patients: a cohort study of 565 patients. J Crit Care. 2017;41:9–15. https://doi.org/10.1016/j.jcrc.2017.04.040.
8. Zahmatkeshan M, Serati Z, Freydooni S, Safarpour AR, Esmailnejad A, Haghbin S. Prediction of early liver failure in pediatric patients admitted to intensive care unit. Middle East J Dig Dis. 2019;11(3):141–6. https://doi.org/10.15171/mejdd.2019.140.
9. Jenniskens M, Güiza F, Haghedooren R, et al. Prevalence and prognostic value of abnormal liver test results in critically ill children and the impact of delaying parenteral nutrition*. Pediatr Crit Care Med. 2018;19(12):1120–9. https://doi.org/10.1097/PCC.0000000000001734.
10. Shteyer E, Yatsiv I, Sharkia M, Milgarter E, Granot E. Serum transaminases as a prognostic factor in children post cardiac surgery. Pediatr Int. 2011;53(5):725–8. https://doi.org/10.1111/j.1442-200X.2011.03356.x.
11. Cheung A, Flamm S. Hepatobiliary complications in critically ill patients. Clin Liver Dis. 2019;23(2):221–32. https://doi.org/10.1016/j.cld.2018.12.005.
12. Fuhrmann V, Kneidinger N, Herkner H, et al. Impact of hypoxic hepatitis on mortality in the intensive care unit. Intensive Care Med. 2011;37(8):1302–10. https://doi.org/10.1007/s00134-011-2248-7.

13. Barañano DE, Rao M, Ferris CD, Snyder SH. Biliverdin reductase: a major physiologic cytoprotectant. Proc Natl Acad Sci U S A. 2002;99(25):16093–8. https://doi.org/10.1073/pnas.252626999.
14. Zelenka J, Muchova L, Zelenkova M, et al. Intracellular accumulation of bilirubin as a defense mechanism against increased oxidative stress. Biochimie. 2012;94(8):1821–7. https://doi.org/10.1016/j.biochi.2012.04.026.
15. Matics TJ, Sanchez-Pinto LN. Adaptation and validation of a pediatric sequential organ failure assessment score and evaluation of the sepsis-3 definitions in critically ill children. JAMA Pediatr. 2017;171(10):e172352. https://doi.org/10.1001/jamapediatrics.2017.2352.
16. Graciano AL, Balko JA, Rahn DS, Ahmad N, Giroir BP. The Pediatric Multiple Organ Dysfunction Score (P-MODS): development and validation of an objective scale to measure the severity of multiple organ dysfunction in critically ill children. Crit Care Med. 2005;33(7):1484–91. https://doi.org/10.1097/01.CCM.0000170943.23633.47.
17. Pollack MM, Patel KM, Ruttimann UE. PRISM III: an updated pediatric risk of mortality score. Crit Care Med. 1996;24(5):743–52. https://doi.org/10.1097/00003246-199605000-00004.
18. Vollmar B, Menger MD. The hepatic microcirculation: mechanistic contributions and therapeutic targets in liver injury and repair. Physiol Rev. 2009;89(4):1269–339. https://doi.org/10.1152/physrev.00027.2008.
19. Henrion J. Hypoxic hepatitis. Liver Int. 2012;32(7):1039–52. https://doi.org/10.1111/j.1478-3231.2011.02655.x.
20. Reilly PM, Wilkins KB, Fuh KC, Haglund U, Bulkley GB. The mesenteric hemodynamic response to circulatory shock: an overview. Shock. 2001;15(5):329–43. https://doi.org/10.1097/00024382-200115050-00001.
21. Fuhrmann V, Kneidinger N, Herkner H, et al. Hypoxic hepatitis: underlying conditions and risk factors for mortality in critically ill patients. Intensive Care Med. 2009;35(8):1397–405. https://doi.org/10.1007/s00134-009-1508-2.
22. Birrer R, Takuda Y, Takara T. Hypoxic hepatopathy: pathophysiology and prognosis. Intern Med. 2007;46(14):1063–70. https://doi.org/10.2169/internalmedicine.46.0059.
23. Fuhrmann V, Jäger B, Zubkova A, Drolz A. Hypoxic hepatitis - epidemiology, pathophysiology and clinical management. Wien Klin Wochenschr. 2010;122(5–6):129–39. https://doi.org/10.1007/s00508-010-1357-6.
24. Trilok G, Qing YC, Li-Jun X. Hypoxic hepatitis: a challenging diagnosis. Hepatol Int. 2012;6(4):663–9. https://doi.org/10.1007/s12072-011-9336-1.
25. Waseem N, Chen P-H. Hypoxic hepatitis: a review and clinical update. J Clin Transl Hepatol. 2016;4(3):263–8. https://doi.org/10.14218/JCTH.2016.00022.
26. Kobashi H, Toshimori J, Yamamoto K. Sepsis-associated liver injury: incidence, classification and the clinical significance. Hepatol Res. 2013;43(3):255–66. https://doi.org/10.1111/j.1872-034X.2012.01069.x.
27. Yao Y, Wang D, Yin Y. Advances in sepsis-associated liver dysfunction. Burns Trauma. 2014;2(3):97. https://doi.org/10.4103/2321-3868.132689.
28. Woźnica EA, Inglot M, Woźnica RK, Łysenko L. Liver dysfunction in sepsis. Adv Clin Exp Med. 2018;27(4):547–51. https://doi.org/10.17219/acem/68363.
29. Strnad P, Tacke F, Koch A, Trautwein C. Liver — guardian, modifier and target of sepsis. Nat Rev Gastroenterol Hepatol. 2017;14(1):55–66. https://doi.org/10.1038/nrgastro.2016.168.
30. Jenniskens M, Langouche L, Vanwijngaerden Y-M, Mesotten D, Van den Berghe G. Cholestatic liver (dys)function during sepsis and other critical illnesses. Intensive Care Med. 2016;42(1):16–27. https://doi.org/10.1007/s00134-015-4054-0.
31. Wells ML, Venkatesh SK. Congestive hepatopathy. Abdom Radiol (NY). 2018;43(8):2037–51. https://doi.org/10.1007/s00261-017-1387-x.
32. Komatsu H, Inui A, Kishiki K, et al. Liver disease secondary to congenital heart disease in children. Expert Rev Gastroenterol Hepatol. 2019;13(7):651–66. https://doi.org/10.1080/17474124.2019.1621746.

33. Xanthopoulos A, Starling RC, Kitai T, Triposkiadis F. Heart failure and liver disease: cardiohepatic interactions. JACC Heart Fail. 2019;7(2):87–97. https://doi.org/10.1016/j.jchf.2018.10.007.
34. Seeto RK, Fenn B, Rockey DC. Ischemic hepatitis: clinical presentation and pathogenesis. Am J Med. 2000;109(2):109–13. https://doi.org/10.1016/s0002-9343(00)00461-7.
35. Henrion J, Schapira M, Luwaert R, Colin L, Delannoy A, Heller FR. Hypoxic hepatitis: clinical and hemodynamic study in 142 consecutive cases. Medicine (Baltimore). 2003;82(6):392–406. https://doi.org/10.1097/01.md.0000101573.54295.bd.
36. Lauriti G, Zani A, Aufieri R, et al. Incidence, prevention, and treatment of parenteral nutrition–associated cholestasis and intestinal failure–associated liver disease in infants and children. J Parenter Enter Nutr. 2014;38(1):70–85. https://doi.org/10.1177/0148607113496280.
37. Rangel SJ, Calkins CM, Cowles RA, et al. Parenteral nutrition–associated cholestasis: an American Pediatric Surgical Association outcomes and clinical trials committee systematic review. J Pediatr Surg. 2012;47(1):225–40. https://doi.org/10.1016/j.jpedsurg.2011.10.007.
38. Grau T, Bonet A, Rubio M, et al. Liver dysfunction associated with artificial nutrition in critically ill patients. Crit Care. 2007;11(1):R10. https://doi.org/10.1186/cc5670.
39. Cahova M, Bratova M, Wohl P. Parenteral nutrition-associated liver disease: the role of the gut microbiota. Nutrients. 2017;9(9):987. https://doi.org/10.3390/nu9090987.
40. Madnawat H, Welu AL, Gilbert EJ, et al. Mechanisms of parenteral nutrition–associated liver and gut injury. Nutr Clin Pract. 2020;35(1):63–71. https://doi.org/10.1002/ncp.10461.
41. Bae HJ, Shin SH, Kim E-K, Kim H-S, Cho YS, Gwak HS. Effects of cyclic parenteral nutrition on parenteral nutrition-associated cholestasis in newborns. Asia Pac J Clin Nutr. 2019;28(1):42–8. https://doi.org/10.6133/apjcn.201903_28(1).0007.
42. Orso G, Mandato C, Veropalumbo C, Cecchi N, Garzi A, Vajro P. Pediatric parenteral nutrition-associated liver disease and cholestasis: novel advances in pathomechanisms-based prevention and treatment. Dig Liver Dis. 2016;48(3):215–22. https://doi.org/10.1016/j.dld.2015.11.003.
43. Lam HS, Tam YH, Poon TCW, et al. A double-blind randomised controlled trial of fish oil-based versus soy-based lipid preparations in the treatment of infants with parenteral nutrition-associated cholestasis. Neonatology. 2014;105(4):290–6. https://doi.org/10.1159/000358267.
44. Zimmerman HJ. Drug-induced liver disease. Clin Liver Dis. 2000;4(1):73–96, vi. https://doi.org/10.1016/s1089-3261(05)70097-0.
45. Amin MD, Harpavat S, Leung DH. Drug-induced liver injury in children. Curr Opin Pediatr. 2015;27(5):625–33. https://doi.org/10.1097/MOP.0000000000000264.
46. Molleston JP, Fontana RJ, Lopez MJ, Kleiner DE, Gu J, Chalasani N. Characteristics of idiosyncratic drug-induced liver injury in children: results from the DILIN prospective study. J Pediatr Gastroenterol Nutr. 2011;53(2):182–9. https://doi.org/10.1097/MPG.0b013e31821d6cfd.
47. Sridharan K, Daylami AA, Ajjawi R, Ajooz HAMA. Drug-induced liver injury in critically ill children taking antiepileptic drugs: a retrospective study. Curr Ther Res Clin Exp. 2020;92:100580. https://doi.org/10.1016/j.curtheres.2020.100580.
48. LiverTox: clinical and research information on drug-induced liver injury. National Institute of Diabetes and Digestive and Kidney Diseases; 2012. Accessed June 26, 2020. http://www.ncbi.nlm.nih.gov/books/NBK547852/.
49. Lescot T, Karvellas C, Beaussier M, Magder S. Acquired liver injury in the intensive care unit. Anesthesiology. 2012;117(4):898–904. https://doi.org/10.1097/ALN.0b013e318266c6df.
50. Pollak U, Ruderman T, Borik-Chiger S, Mishaly D, Serraf A, Vardi A. Transfusion-related acute hepatic injury following postoperative platelets administration in pediatric patients undergoing the Fontan procedure. Congenit Heart Dis. 2019;14(6):968–77. https://doi.org/10.1111/chd.12825.
51. Nachnani JS, Hamid F, Pandya P, Clarkston W, Alba LM. Transfusion-related acute hepatic enzyme elevation: a new disease entity? Eur J Gastroenterol Hepatol. 2010;22(3):378. https://doi.org/10.1097/MEG.0b013e3283279681.

52. Gudnason HO, Björnsson ES. Secondary sclerosing cholangitis in critically ill patients: current perspectives. Clin Exp Gastroenterol. 2017;10:105–11. https://doi.org/10.2147/CEG.S115518.
53. Martins P, Verdelho MM. Secondary Sclerosing cholangitis in critically ill patients: an underdiagnosed entity. GE Port J Gastroenterol. 2020;27(2):103–14. https://doi.org/10.1159/000501405.
54. Garland JS, Werlin SL, Rice TB. Ischemic hepatitis in children: diagnosis and clinical course. Crit Care Med. 1988;16(12):1209–12. https://doi.org/10.1097/00003246-198812000-00006.
55. Fuhrmann V, Madl C, Mueller C, et al. Hepatopulmonary syndrome in patients with hypoxic hepatitis. Gastroenterology. 2006;131(1):69–75. https://doi.org/10.1053/j.gastro.2006.04.014.
56. Drolz A, Horvatits T, Michl B, et al. Statin therapy is associated with reduced incidence of hypoxic hepatitis in critically ill patients. J Hepatol. 2014;60(6):1187–93. https://doi.org/10.1016/j.jhep.2014.01.019.
57. Jenniskens M, Langouche L, Van den Berghe G. Cholestatic alterations in the critically ill: some new light on an old problem. Chest. 2018;153(3):733–43. https://doi.org/10.1016/j.chest.2017.08.018.
58. Brienza N, Dalfino L, Cinnella G, Diele C, Bruno F, Fiore T. Jaundice in critical illness: promoting factors of a concealed reality. Intensive Care Med. 2006;32(2):267–74. https://doi.org/10.1007/s00134-005-0023-3.
59. Newsome PN, Cramb R, Davison SM, et al. Guidelines on the management of abnormal liver blood tests. Gut. 2018;67(1):6–19. https://doi.org/10.1136/gutjnl-2017-314924.
60. Horvatits T, Drolz A, Rutter K, et al. Circulating bile acids predict outcome in critically ill patients. Ann Intensive Care. 2017;7(1):48. https://doi.org/10.1186/s13613-017-0272-7.
61. Manzotti C, Casazza G, Stimac T, Nikolova D, Gluud C. Total serum bile acids or serum bile acid profile, or both, for the diagnosis of intrahepatic cholestasis of pregnancy. Cochrane Database Syst Rev. 2019;7:CD012546. https://doi.org/10.1002/14651858.CD012546.pub2.
62. Halle BM, Poulsen TD, Pedersen HP. Indocyanine green plasma disappearance rate as dynamic liver function test in critically ill patients. Acta Anaesthesiol Scand. 2014;58(10):1214–9. https://doi.org/10.1111/aas.12406.
63. Sakka SG. Assessing liver function. Curr Opin Crit Care. 2007;13(2):207–14. https://doi.org/10.1097/MCC.0b013e328012b268.
64. Kortgen A, Paxian M, Werth M, et al. Prospective assessment of hepatic function and mechanisms of dysfunction in the critically ill. Shock. 2009;32(4):358–65. https://doi.org/10.1097/SHK.0b013e31819d8204.
65. Kimura S, Yoshioka T, Shibuya M, Sakano T, Tanaka R, Matsuyama S. Indocyanine green elimination rate detects hepatocellular dysfunction early in septic shock and correlates with survival. Crit Care Med. 2001;29(6):1159–63. https://doi.org/10.1097/00003246-200106000-00014.
66. Sakka SG, Reinhart K, Meier-Hellmann A. Prognostic value of the indocyanine green plasma disappearance rate in critically ill patients. Chest. 2002;122(5):1715–20. https://doi.org/10.1378/chest.122.5.1715.
67. Horvatits T, Kneidinger N, Drolz A, et al. Prognostic impact of ICG-PDR in patients with hypoxic hepatitis. Ann Intensive Care. 2015;5(1):47. https://doi.org/10.1186/s13613-015-0092-6.
68. Vos JJ, Wietasch JKG, Absalom AR, Hendriks HGD, Scheeren TWL. Green light for liver function monitoring using indocyanine green? An overview of current clinical applications. Anaesthesia. 2014;69(12):1364–76. https://doi.org/10.1111/anae.12755.
69. Koch A, Horn A, Dückers H, et al. Increased liver stiffness denotes hepatic dysfunction and mortality risk in critically ill non-cirrhotic patients at a medical ICU. Crit Care. 2011;15(6):R266. https://doi.org/10.1186/cc10543.
70. Fink T, Heymann P, Taha-Melitz S, et al. Dobutamine pretreatment improves survival, liver function, and hepatic microcirculation after polymicrobial sepsis in rat. Shock. 2013;40(2):129–35. https://doi.org/10.1097/SHK.0b013e31829c361d.

71. Raddatz A, Kubulus D, Winning J, et al. Dobutamine improves liver function after hemorrhagic shock through induction of heme oxygenase-1. Am J Respir Crit Care Med. 2006;174(2):198–207. https://doi.org/10.1164/rccm.200508-1221OC.
72. Simić D, Milojević I, Bogićević D, et al. Preventive effect of ursodeoxycholic acid on parenteral nutrition-associated liver disease in infants. Srp Arh Celok Lek. 2014;142(3-4):184–8. https://doi.org/10.2298/sarh1404184s.
73. Drolz A, Horvatits T, Roedl K, et al. Outcome and features of acute kidney injury complicating hypoxic hepatitis at the medical intensive care unit. Ann Intensive Care. 2016;6(1):61. https://doi.org/10.1186/s13613-016-0162-4.
74. El Banayosy A. First use of the Molecular Adsorbent Recirculating System technique on patients with hypoxic liver failure after cardiogenic shock. ASAIO J. 2004;50(4):332–7.
75. Falkensteiner C, Kortgen A, Leonhardt J, Bauer M, Sponholz C. Comparison of the albumin dialysis devices molecular adsorbent recirculating system and ADVanced organ support in critically ill patients with liver failure - a retrospective analysis. Ther Apher Dial. 2021;25:225–36. https://doi.org/10.1111/1744-9987.13533.
76. Polson J, Lee WM. AASLD position paper: the management of acute liver failure. Hepatology. 2005;41(5):1179–97. https://doi.org/10.1002/hep.20703.
77. George R, Stevens A, Berkenbosch JW, Turpin J, Tobias J. Ursodeoxycholic acid in the treatment of cholestasis and hyperbilirubinemia in pediatric intensive care unit patients. South Med J. 2002;95(11):1276–9.
78. Kramer L, Stauber R, Lenz K, Schusterschitz N, Trauner M, Joannidis M. A randomized controlled multicenter trial of high dose ursodesoxycholic acid versus placebo in sepsis-assoicated cholestasis. Z Für Gastroenterol. 2010;48(5):P8. https://doi.org/10.1055/s-0030-1254616.
79. Lee WM, Hynan LS, Rossaro L, et al. Intravenous N-acetylcysteine improves transplant-free survival in early stage non-acetaminophen acute liver failure. Gastroenterology. 2009;137(3):856–864.e1. https://doi.org/10.1053/j.gastro.2009.06.006.
80. Singh S, Hynan LS, Lee WM, Acute Liver Failure Study Group. Improvements in hepatic serological biomarkers are associated with clinical benefit of intravenous N-acetylcysteine in early stage non-acetaminophen acute liver failure. Dig Dis Sci. 2013;58(5):1397–402. https://doi.org/10.1007/s10620-012-2512-x.

Acute Liver Failure

Fernando Alvarez and Philippe Jouvet

Acute liver failure is characterized by a rapid deterioration in liver functions, including mainly a coagulopathy and changes in the mental status, leading to an encephalopathy. Acute liver failure is a life-threatening critical condition that occurs rarely, in patients without pre-existing liver disease. This severe liver injury can be reversible, and substantial advances in the treatment have remarkably improved survival in recent years.

Definition

The Paediatric Acute Liver Failure (PALF) Group proposed the following criteria for the diagnosis of acute liver failure: (1) children with no known evidence of chronic liver disease, (2) biochemical evidence of acute liver injury, and (3) hepatic-based coagulopathy defined as a prothrombin time (PT) $\geq$15 s or INR $\geq$1.5 not corrected by Vitamin K in the presence of clinical hepatic encephalopathy (HE) or a PT $\geq$20 s or INR $\geq$2.0 regardless of the presence or absence of clinical HE [1].

Fulminant and subfulminant liver failure were the original terms used to define acute liver failure according to the delay between first symptoms or signs and onset of the encephalopathy. Fulminant hepatic failure requires the onset of encephalopathy in the first 2 weeks, and subfulminant hepatic failure in between 2 and 12 weeks

F. Alvarez
Division of Gastroenterology, Hepatology & Nutrition, Department of Pediatrics of Sainte Justine Hospital, University of Montreal, Montréal, QC, Canada
e-mail: fernando.alvarez@umontreal.ca

P. Jouvet (✉)
Pediatric Intensive Care Unit - Department of Pediatrics of Sainte Justine Hospital, University of Montreal, Montréal, QC, Canada
e-mail: philippe.jouvet.med@ssss.gouv.qc.ca

P. Jouvet, F. Alvarez (eds.), *Liver Diseases in the Pediatric Intensive Care Unit*,
https://doi.org/10.1007/978-3-030-79132-2_2

from the beginning of symptoms and signs of hepatic failure, frequently jaundice. More recently, severe liver injury was considered as hyperacute when encephalopathy is diagnosed in the first week, acute between 8 and 28 days, and subacute between 5 and 12 weeks. Patients with hyperacute failure frequently develop cerebral oedema, but they have good chances of survival. Patients with acute liver failure also show high incidence of cerebral oedema, but a poorer prognosis without liver transplantation; patients with subacute liver failure have a poor prognosis of liver regeneration, even if they have a low incidence of cerebral oedema [2].

Aetiologies of Acute Liver Failure in Newborn and Infants (Tables 1 and 2)

In a study by the Paediatric Acute Liver Failure group, in 148 children younger than 90 days of life, the most frequent cause of liver failure was indeterminate in 38%, secondary to an alloimmune foetal hepatitis in 13.6%, and due to herpes simplex

Table 1 Aetiologies of severe acute liver failure according to patient's age

Age	Diseases
Newborns (<1 month of age)	Viral hepatitis: Herpes, echovirus, coxsacke, adenovirus Inherited disease: Galactosemia, mitochondriopathies, PFIC type 2, bile acid metabolism defects Foetal (gestational) alloimmune hepatitis Shock – severe hypoxia Vascular – peliosis hepatis
Infants (between 1 month and 1 year of age)	Viral hepatitis: Hepatitis A virus, Hepatitis B virus, Hepatitis E virus, Parvovirus, Adenovirus Inherited diseases: Tyrosinemia, fructosaemia, mitochondriopathies, PFIC type 2, bile acid metabolism defects Drug toxicity: Acetaminophen, valproic acid Hemophagocytic/lymphohistiocytose Vascular – peliosis hepatis Shock – severe hypoxia Malignancy Giant cell hepatitis with immune-mediated haemolytic anaemia Indeterminate hepatitis
Children (older than 1 year of age)	Viral hepatitis: Hepatitis A virus, Hepatitis B virus, Hepatitis E virus, Epstein-Barr virus Drug toxicity: Acetaminophen*, valproic acid (other anticonvulsant agents) Autoimmune hepatitis type 1 and type 2 Giant cell hepatitis with immune mediated haemolytic anaemia Vascular: Veno-occlusive disease, Budd-Chiari Haemophagocytic lymphohistiocytose Inherited diseases: Wilson's disease Indeterminate hepatitis Mushroom (amanita phalloides) intoxication *Acetaminophen toxicity is particularly observed in adolescents

PFIC type 2 Progressive familial intrahepatic cholestasis type 2

Table 2 Causes of acute liver failure and frequency (number of +) by age

Infections	**<12 m**	**>12 m**
HSV 1 and 2	++	+
HBV(+HDV)	++	+++
HEV	±	+++
HAV	±	+++
Rubeola	+	–
Syphilis	+	–
EBV	–	–
CMV	+	–
Enterovirus	++	–
Parvovirus B19	+	+
Adenovirus	+	+
Arbovirus	–	+
Metabolic	**<12 m**	**>12 m**
Tyrosinemia	++	+
Galactosaemia	++	–
Fructosaemia	++	–
OTC[a]	+	–
CPS[b]	+	–
Wilson disease	–	+++
Inborn errors BA[c] metabolism	+	–
Alpers	–	+
Mitochondria	++	–
Toxic		
Acetaminophen	±	+++
Mushroom	–	++
Anaesthetics	–	+
Antibiotics	–	++
Valproic acid	–	+
Isoniazid	–	±
Other	+	++
Immune related	**<12 m**	**>12 m**
Alloimmune	+++	–
AIH	±	+++
Giant cell hepatitis and AHA[d]	++	+
Vascular	**<12 m**	**>12 m**
Hypoxia/shock	++	+
Venocclusive	+	+
Budd-Chiari	–	+
Peliose	+	±
Haematological	**<12 m**	**>12 m**

(continued)

Table 2 (continued)

Haemophagocytosis	++	+
Leukaemia	+	+
Lymphome	−	+

[a]OTC Ornithine transcarbamylase deficiency
[b]CPS Carbamoyl phosphate synthetase deficiency
[c]BA Bile acids
[d]AHA Autoimmune haemolytic anaemia
HSV herpes simplex virus, *HA(B,D,E)V* hepatitis A(B,D,E) virus, *EBV* Ebstein Barr Virus, *CMV* Cytomegalovirus, *AIH* Allo Immune hepatitis.

infection in 12.8% of them. Other viral infections leading to hepatic failure at this age were enterovirus (echovirus, Coxackie virus) and cytomegalovirus (mostly severe congenital cases). Metabolic diseases were also reported, such as galactosaemia (8%), mitochondrial diseases including respiratory chain defects (5.4%), tyrosinaemia and Niemann-Pick type C (2% each), and urea cycle defects (1.4%). Other aetiologies that have also been reported were: shock (4%), haemophagocytic syndrome (2.7%), septicaemia (1.4%), hemangioendothelioma (1.4%) [3]. Sixty percent of these infants survived spontaneously and 40% were transplanted or died. Those with viral infection showed a higher risk of death. Patients showed lower mean increase of ALT than older children in acute liver failure, being the increase higher in those with viral infections (mean 618 IU/l) than those with indeterminate cause (109 IU/l), and foetal alloimmune hepatitis that showed ALT serum levels close to normal values (mean 35 IU/l). Thus, ALT serum levels should be considered in the differential diagnosis of the cause of acute liver failure [3, 4].

A large series of infants from Bicêtre Hospital showed that metabolic disorders were the main cause of acute liver failure (42.5%), followed by foetal alloimmune hepatitis (16.2%), indeterminate hepatitis (16.2%), viral hepatitis (15%), and other causes (10%) [5].

Similar results were shown in a work from the King's College of London, being in this centre the foetal alloimmune hepatitis the most frequent aetiology of acute liver failure in children under the age of 1 year (26%), and the cause of this disorder in 40% of newborns. Viral infections were found in 25% of newborns, and in 21.5% of children less than 1 year of age. Interestingly, haematological malignancies were diagnosed in 10% of children under the age of 1 year. As it was previously published, viral infections at this age had the worst prognosis [6, 7].

Metabolic diseases and foetal alloimmune hepatitis are the main cause of acute liver failure in children less than 1 year old.

Some metabolic diseases have no indication of liver transplantation due to their reversibility under specific treatment or their multiorgan involvement.

Metabolic Diseases

Galactosaemia-induced liver failure onset occurs in the first month of life, rarely afterward, usually presenting with a septicaemia due to Gram negative infection, most frequently by E coli. First symptoms and signs are abdominal distension, vomiting, and loss of appetite, as well as fever, jaundice, and a firm hepatomegaly. Biochemical tests show the frequent presence of coagulopathy, hypoglycaemia, and hyperbirubinaemia, the latter could be aggravated by a haemolytic anaemia. This clinical picture is quite characteristic of galactosaemia, and the presence of punctate cataracts practically establish the diagnosis, that is confirmed by the increase of galactose-1-phosphate and other galactose metabolites in serum and urine, dosage in erythrocytes of the galactose-1-phosphate uridyl transferase or by genetic studies of its gene [8].

Tyrosinaemia, presents as an acute liver failure in infants from the second month of life, and rarely after 1 year of age. At onset a nodular liver is already observed at the ultrasound. Hepatic failure concerns mainly the protein synthesis function of hepatocytes, and in most cases is reversible by treatment with Nitisinone (NTBC) [9].

Fructosaemia, the result of a catalytic deficiency of aldolase B in the liver, very rarely present as an acute liver failure. In these infants, symptoms appear after the exposition to fructose or sucrose, in young babies receiving a high load of these carbohydrates. Symptoms and signs are: vomiting, diarrhoea, abdominal distension, and pain. Hepatomegaly is recorded, and biochemical tests show hypophosphataemia, hypoglycaemia, hyperlactacidaemia, and hyperuricaemia [10].

Mitochondrial disorders can present with acute liver failure early in life. These defects of the oxidative phosphorylation rarely show exclusively liver-related symptoms and signs; in most cases other organs are affected. Symptoms as diarrhoea, seizures, hypotonia, and other neurological manifestations are frequently present at onset. Lactate/pyruvate molar ratios and ketone body ratios are of help in the suspicion of a mitochondrial bioenergetics defect [11–14].

Defects in the TRMU gene encoding the mitochondrial tRNA-specific 2-thiouridylase were found in infants with acute liver failure. It is characterized by a combined defect of respiratory chain complexes without mitochondrial DNA depletion. Some children can recover spontaneously in few months, whereas others can die during the episode [15]. A case received a liver transplant at CHU-Sainte Justine, now at the age of 5 years, is showing a stable development delay, and increase of serum creatine kinase levels without signs of myopathy. Deficiency of different proteins intervening in the intracellular trafficking, as those coded by the SCYL1 and the NBAS genes, can also be responsible for recurrent acute liver failure during febrile infectious episodes. In addition, these deficiencies are associated with neurological or multisystemic phenotypes [16, 17].

Mitochondrial fatty acid oxidation defects can show signs of liver dysfunction, as hypoketotic hypoglycaemia, and frequently present as fasting-induced vomiting. Hypotonia and other signs of myopathy are consequently found [18].

Other rare causes of acute liver failure in these very young patients could be: some inborn errors of bile acid metabolism and progressive familial intrahepatic cholestasis type 2.

Recently, some cases of cholestasis and hepatic failure have been described, associated to a pyruvate kinase deficiency. Cholestasis onset is observed early after birth, showing normal serum GGT levels, and liver failure develops in between the first and fourth month of life. The pyruvate kinase deficiency is responsible for severe haemolysis, and also affects the activity of this enzyme in the liver, producing a decrease in energy synthesis in hepatocytes [19, 20].

Urea cycle disorders can present early in life as an acute liver failure. The main diseases in this group are: (1) Hyperornithinaemia-Hyperammoniaemia-Homocitrullinuria syndrome produced by the deficiency of the ornithine carrier in the inner mitochondria membrane, coded by the SLC25A15 gene; and enzyme deficiencies as (2) Ornithine transcarbamylase deficiency, the gene coding for this enzyme located in the X chromosome; (3) Carbamylphosphate synthetase 1 deficiency; (4) Argininosuccinate synthetase deficiency; (5) Argininosuccinate lyase; and (6) Arginase 1 deficiency. Deficiency of the latter three enzymes is transmitted in an autosomal recessive manner. Early acute onset in children with urea cycle disorders presents tachypnea, respiratory alkalosis, gastrointestinal symptoms as vomiting and poor appetite, and acute encephalopathy characterized by seizures, lethargy, confusion, or coma. Such symptoms are associated in some cases to increase in serum aminotransferases, sometimes massively increased, and signs of coagulopathy [21, 22].

Indeterminate Hepatitis

Indeterminate hepatitis is infrequent in newborns and infants; but when it occurs the final outcome is as unfavourable as in older children. In some cohorts from the USA, indeterminate hepatitis is more frequently reported than in European ones; however, testing for viruses in the former was not always optimal in all centres [23]. Strategies improving diagnostic testing have recently reduced the percentage of indeterminate hepatitis cases in US centres [24].

Viral Infections

Enteroviruses and herpes simplex virus are the most frequently found in the neonatal period, and among enteroviruses the Coxsackievirus B, and Echoviruses 3, 21, 30, 33. Patients with enterovirus infection can recover spontaneously or need a liver transplant; no available data help in the decision between wait or proceed with a liver transplantation at this age. Patients with suspected or confirmed Herpes Simplex infection should receive intravenous acyclovir. In children showing a spontaneous recovery after enterovirus hepatitis, atrophy of part of the liver can be observed as a sequel of the severe parenchymal injury.

Hepatitis B infection by vertical transmission or blood derivatives (currently exceptional in developed countries) can present as an acute liver failure after an incubation time between 70 and 150 days of life [25].

Haemophagocytic Lymphohistiocytosis (HLH)

HLH most frequently affects infants, but it is also observed in children and adolescents. The disease can be sporadic or the result of a genetic defect (familial). Many of the so-called sporadic cases show in effect some heterozygous defects or double heterozygous; in general presenting at older age for the single heterozygous children [26]. Triggers of the disease are variable, but infections are the most frequent ones. In some systemic inflammatory diseases a "Macrophagic Activation Syndrome" can occur, as described in patients with juvenile idiopathic arthritis.

In HLH the tissue destruction, an "excessive" inflammation, and abnormal immune activation are the consequence of a deficiency in the down-regulation of activated macrophages and lymphocytes. Haemophagocytosis is characterized by the presence of white blood cells, red blood cells, and platelets in macrophages cytoplasm; however, such feature is sometimes difficult to find in bone marrow, lymph nodes, spleen, or liver of patients with HLH.

Patients with HLH and liver failure show some clinical and laboratory differences when compared with children having a liver damage, but of indeterminate aetiology. Pleural effusion, splenomegaly, and fever, as well as anaemia, thrombocytopenia, and initial hypoalbuminaemia were more frequent, and CRP and serum triglycerides higher in patients with liver failure is associated to HLH. Hepatomegaly, liver enzymes, white blood cells, and coagulation profile did not show significant differences [27].

Foetal Alloimmune Hepatitis

Foetal or gestational alloimmune hepatitis, previously called neonatal haemochromatosis, is characterized by a severe foetal-neonatal liver injury leading to early onset hepatic failure in the post-natal period. Previous immunized mothers develop antibodies against foetal hepatocyte antigens, IgG pass through the placenta into the foetal blood stream, and bind to hepatocytes surfaces fixing complement and inducing cell damage. Detection of the Membrane Attack Complex (MAC- form by Complement 5b-9) on cell surfaces during liver biopsy is of great help in the diagnosis of the disease. Antecedents of previous spontaneous abortions or newborns with liver disease ("idiopathic neonatal cholestasis") are frequently recorded. In severe cases death occurs in foetal life, with or without preceding evidence of foetal distress [28].

Foetal liver failure, in severe cases, leads to a low production of hepcidin, the hormone, secreted by the liver, responsible for regulating the absorption of the iron in the intestine and its passage through the placenta. Unregulated iron passage at the placenta level leads to foetal siderosis implicating the liver and extra-hepatic tissues, as observed in most newborns with foetal alloimmune hepatitis. Diagnosis can be highly suspected by the presence of iron deposition in salivary gland biopsies in more than 60% of cases. Newborns with foetal alloimmune hepatitis but without iron overload have also been described [29]. In standard blood tests the more helpful iron index for the suspicion of the disease is a high value of transferrin binding saturation, associated with an excess of non-transferrin-bound iron, even in cases with a transferrin binding capacity in or close to normal values [30].

Maternal treatment with antenatal intravenous immunoglobulin infusions (1 g/kg weekly of immunoglobulins from the week 18th of gestation) avoids the development of severe liver failure, in some children only mild signs of transient hepatitis are observed [31]. In newborns with a foetal alloimmune hepatitis, exchange transfusion and intravenous immunoglobulins improve outcome, reducing also the need for a liver transplantation [32].

Giant Cell Hepatitis with Autoimmune Haemolytic Anaemia

Usually, the onset of this disorder occurs in the two first years of life, mean age 1 year, less frequently in older children. Autoimmune haemolytic anaemia precedes or overlaps with the liver disease. No hyper-IgG or particular circulating autoantibodies are found at the onset. High levels of serum ALT are recorded. Immunosuppressive treatment should be rapidly administered, trying to avoid liver transplantation. Severe recurrence of the disease in the transplanted liver is almost the rule [33–35].

Vascular Disorders/Decrease in Liver Perfusion

Acute or subacute drop in liver perfusion can produce jaundice, hepatomegaly, and when portal hypertension develops, rapid development of ascites. Spontaneous evolution is variable, either toward regression or progression of the liver failure. Laboratory results show an increase of bilirubin and serum aminotransferases at variable levels, hypoalbuminaemia, and abnormal coagulation tests.

Peliosis hepatitis onset occurs in the great majority on patients under the age of 18 months, with rare exceptions. In general this disorder is associated with other extra-hepatic diseases or bacterial infections. A neonatal case was described, secondary to ingestion of fenvalerate, an insecticide, by the mother drinking contaminated green tea during pregnancy [36].

Veno-occlussive disease (sinusoidal occlusion) was described in a newborn whose mother drank a Jamaican herbal tea contaminated with pyrrolizidine. Young children receiving infusions from similar herbs containing the same alkaloid have also developed the disease.

Liver failure secondary to a shock leading to severe liver hypoxia has been described in the peri-natal period. However, it can also occur at any time, mainly in children with severe cardiopathy, in particular in the post-operatory period of reparation surgery.

Etiologies of Acute Liver Failure in Children (Tables 1 and 2)

Causes are variable in different regions of the world, being mainly drug-induced or so-called indeterminate in the industrialized world and secondary to viral infections in the less industrialized world, mainly due to hepatitis A, B, or E. Other causes with universal distribution are: metabolic (ex; Wilson disease), autoimmune hepatitis, or intoxication with mushrooms (*amanita phalloides*).

The Pediatric Acute Liver Failure (PALF) study group showed that in USA, the main causes of acute liver failure were: indeterminate hepatitis (49%), acetaminophen toxicity (14%), mainly in older children/adolescents, followed by autoimmune hepatitis (6%), and viral infections (6%) [1]. The very high percentage of indeterminate hepatitis could also be explained by the incomplete testing for viruses or paracetamol levels; thus some viral or paracetamol causes of acute liver failure are underdiagnosed [23, 24]. Similar numbers could be found in European cohorts, with a slightly higher prevalence of paracetamol intoxication in series from the United Kingdom [6].

Indeterminate Hepatitis

Indeterminate hepatitis is the most frequent cause of acute liver failure in children of more than 1 year old. Usually, it develops as a severe non-regenerative liver injury, in which encephalopathy occurs late in the evolution. Prognosis of this disorder is worse than in other known causes of liver failure. In some patients, rescue therapy with immunosuppressive drugs could be successfully led to liver recovery [37].

Most cases of acute liver failure of indeterminate etiology present signs of hyperinflammatory state, opening the possibility of treatment with immunosuppressive drugs [38, 39].

> Indeterminate hepatitis is the main cause of acute liver failure in children older than 1 year of age.

> In children with indeterminate hepatitis a bone marrow aplasia can complicate the clinical picture.

Viral Infections

The most frequent viral infection complicated with acute liver failure in children are: hepatitis A, and B viruses, and also hepatitis E virus genotypes 1 and 2 in some non-industrialized countries. In recent years the incidence of hepatitis A and B virus became very low in industrialized countries due to availability of vaccines; in these countries very rare cases of Hepatitis E Virus genotype 3-induced acute liver failure were reported. Other viruses, even if much less frequent, can be responsible for an acute liver failure as: Epstein Barr virus, and Herpes Simplex, and rarely Adenovirus, Parvovirus, Ebola virus, Dengue virus, Toga virus. Parvovirus infection inducing an acute liver failure is more frequent in children under the age of 5 years, showing low bilirubin levels, and recovering rapidly from the hepatic injury [40]. However, Parvovirus-induced liver failure was also described in older patients needing a liver transplant followed by a Bone Marrow Transplantation [41].

Drugs

As in other causes of severe acute hepatic failure, signs of hepatocellular injury are high serum levels of aminotransferases, and of bilirubin without other signs of cholestasis (low alkaline phosphatase and gamma-glutamyl transferase). Drugs can induce severe liver failure by two different mechanisms: direct toxicity or immune-mediated reactivity (idiosyncratic reaction).

- *Careful questioning of patients and parents on drugs/xenobiotics exposure must always be done*

Idiosyncratic-drug induced liver injury occurs after a certain delay from the exposition to the drug, and are of variable degree from mild to severe. Reactive metabolites of a xenobiotic covalently bind to hepatocytes proteins generate an immune response, the immune reactivity against the complex depends on the immune tolerance level in a particular individual [42].

Paracetamol/Acetaminophen

The most common drug associated with liver failure is paracetamol/acetaminophen, mainly around adolescence, due to the deliberated ingestion of high amounts of this medication. Acetaminophen adducts are detected in most intoxicated patients, as well in others that ingested such medication during the course of an acute hepatitis of another cause. The role and contribution of such adducts in the hepatic failure is unknown [43]. Acetamoniphen metabolism produces a reactive metabolite (N-acetyl-p-benzoquinone) that covalently binds to hepatocyte proteins, and is detoxified by gluthatione. Once gluthatione is depleted the covalent reactive metabolite is found in the liver. N-acetylcysteine is an antidote for acetamoniphen toxicity binding the reactive metabolite and increasing the synthesis of gluthatione. CYP2E1 is the major cause of the formation of reactive metabolites, even if CYP1A2 and 3A also contribute. More than 90 mg/kg in children should be considered as toxic. After a massive overdose of acetaminophen the Rumack-Matthew normogram is a reliable tool to establish toxic levels according to the time from the ingestion, after 24 h of the overdose the diagnosis can be challenging. However, an increase of serum aminotransferases is a marker of liver toxicity at that time. Acetaminophen protein adducts serum levels are good markers of liver injury, with a good correlation with aminotransferases serum levels. Lactic acidosis can occur early at very high concentrations of paracetamol by inhibition of electron transfer in the mitochondrial respiratory chain resulting in inhibition of aerobic respiration. This precedes liver cellular injury by several hours. The second scenario in which lactic acidosis can occur is later in the course of paracetamol poisoning as a consequence of established liver failure [44].

Signs of liver injury show a peak in between the third and the fourth day after acetaminophen excessive ingestion, associated with 40% of cases to renal injury, mainly tubular necrosis. Usually bilirubin remains relatively low, when compared to other causes of acute liver failure.

In paracetamol/acetaminophen intoxication, N'Acetylcysteine should be started as soon as possible.

Isoniazid

Increase of serum aminotransferase levels is common and usually transient in patients taking isoniazid. However, isoniazid can cause an acute liver failure; thus when jaundice is present the drug should be immediately stopped. Such jaundice is indicating a high risk of acute liver failure if the administration of the drug is continued. Toxicity is more frequent in patients with higher CYP2E1 activity or in those with a chronic liver disease [45].

Volatile Anaesthetic Agents (Halothane, Desflurane, Enflurane, Isoflurane, and Sevoflurane)

Halothane is the best known, and its mechanism of toxicity appears to be immune related. For other volatile anaesthetic drugs the mechanism of liver injury is less well known, and the incidence rare.

Anticonvulsant Agents: Phenytoin, Carbamazepine, Valproic acid, and Some of the Newer Anticonvulsants

Carbamazepine is responsible for idiosyncratic liver injury, even if it is frequently observed; fulminant hepatic failure requiring a liver transplant is a rare complication. Phenytoin, can also provoke an idiosyncratic liver damage, in general mild and regressing rapidly after withdrawal of the medication, and very rarely progressing to severe acute liver injury. Among these drugs the valproic acid is the most frequently associated with fulminant liver failure. Even if most cases occur during the first 6 months of therapy, late severe liver failure has been described. Valproic acid can unmask latent heterozygous OTC deficiency, leading to hyperammoniaemia and coma, and such severe outcome is also observed in patients with Alpert disease, associated with mitochondrial permeability transition pore opening-dependent apoptotic sensitivity [46]. Risk of hepatic failure is higher in younger patients receiving polytherapy with other antiepileptic drugs.

Other Drugs

Amoxicillin/clavulanate association is responsible mainly for cholestasis; however, some cases of liver failure have been recorded in patients receiving such medication.

Toxics

Increased usage of dietary/herbal supplements throughout the world could be toxic for the liver, producing in rare cases an acute liver failure, even if more frequent in adults than in children.

Mushrooms intoxication, mainly with *amanita phalloides*, is much more frequent in people from countries or regions with a tradition of collecting and eating wild mushrooms. Abdominal pain, nausea, vomiting, and watery diarrhoea are frequently the initial symptoms, followed by symptoms and signs of liver failure [47].

Autoimmune

Autoimmune hepatitis types 1 and 2 can present as severe acute liver failure in around 5% of cases, most of these cases could be classified as subfulminant or subacute. Children with autoimmune hepatitis type 2 usually develop severe liver failure at younger age than those with autoimmune hepatitis type 1 [48–50]. Treatment by immunosuppressive drugs can be lifesaving in few cases; most would need a liver transplantation. High doses immunosuppression previous to the liver transplant can increase the risk of post-transplant infections. Corticosteroids can induce gluconeogenesis and increase ammonia levels; administration of proteins should be carefully controlled [51].

Metabolic

Wilson can be considered in the differential diagnosis of an acute liver failure after the age of 4 years. Some particular features distinguish Wilson disease from other causes of acute liver failure. In around half of the patients a Kayser-Fleischer ring can be detectable. The presence of a Coombs negative haemolytic anaemia is almost the rule. Oxidation of membrane phospholipids occurs in the red cells plasma membranes, secondary to Cu^{++} release by necrosis or apoptosis of hepatocytes. Serum ALT levels correlate with haemoglobin concentrations. In presence of the anaemia, a high AST/ALT ratio is observed [52].

Patients with severe acute onset of Wilson disease can recover under treatment with Cu^{++} chelators [53]. The indication of a liver transplant is difficult, needing an individual approach, until a reliable prognostic score would be available [54].

Hematological Disorders

Malignant infiltration of the liver can be responsible for liver failure, usually presenting as an acute onset. In paediatric patients, the more frequent malignancies causing severe liver injury are leukaemia and lymphoma. Even if rare, these conditions should be considered before an indication of a liver transplant; a liver biopsy could be indicated. Fatigue and fever followed by jaundice are frequent at onset [55].

Different types of leukaemia and lymphomas were reported as responsible for acute liver failure [56], acute lymphoblastic of pre-B type, myeloblastic, large B-cell lymphoma, hepatosplenic $\gamma\delta$ T-cell lymphoma [57–60].

Haemophagocytic lymphohystiocytosis has mainly been present in infants; however, it can also be observed in older children, with similar clinical features.

Vascular Disorders

Budd-Chiari syndrome is usually considered as a chronic liver disease produced by the outflow obstruction of the hepatic veins; however, some cases can present in a fulminant form. Jaundice and rapid forming ascites are the main signs of the disease.

Veno-occlusive or sinusoidal obstructive disease in children is most frequently the complication of high doses of chemotherapy administered as myeloablative conditioning. Defibrotide is frequently used in the prevention and treatment of this complication. Hepatic veno-occlusive disease has also been observed in patients with immunodeficiency associated to mutations of the gene coding for Sp110 [61].

Pyrrolizidine alkaloids can produce a veno-occlusive disease at any time in life; such alkaloid could be present in plants contaminating different cultures, producing several cases of the disease in the population ingesting such contaminated cereals.

An episode of shock of any cause can be responsible for severe liver injury, secondary to liver hypoperfusion; the splanchnic system is the first suffering vasoconstriction in hypovolemic situations. Generally, spontaneous recovery occurs in most of these cases.

Clinical Presentation

The clinical symptoms and signs of severe hepatic failure vary according to the cause, and the age of patients. The presence or absence of jaundice can help in the differential diagnosis of a toxic liver injury. Paracetamol/Acetaminophen-induced liver failure rarely show an increase of serum bilirubin levels. Such sign is also important in the differential diagnosis of metabolic diseases in infants; as an example, serum bilirubin levels are usually normal or close to normal in children with tyrosinaemia presenting as a liver failure. In causes inducing apoptosis or necrosis of hepatocytes, disorganization of the lobule structure lead to increase in serum bilirubin levels.

In newborns, failure to thrive, vomiting, or signs of compromise of multiple organs as in mitochondrial diseases, are observed at the presentation of metabolic diseases. In older children, nausea, vomiting, and anorexia are frequent.

Bleeding, hypoglycaemia leading to seizures, and encephalopathy can be recorded at onset in the most severe cases or during the follow-up. Encephalopathy is of difficult diagnosis in newborn and infants, changes in the normal behaviour could be the only symptom. In children symptoms and signs are similar to those described in adults and can be evaluated using the four stage liver encephalopathy scale (see chapter Liver Failure and Brain).

Electroencephalogram (EEG) is used to detect covert HE, for example when clinical exam is disturbed by sedative drugs, to detect seizures, or to monitor the severity of liver encephalopathy regardless of patient cooperation, especially in infants.

Several factors can exacerbate hepatic encephalopathy including hypovolaemia-induced or not by diuretics, increase nitrogen intake and/or endogenous protein catabolism via ammonia level increase (Fig. 1), electrolytes disorders (hyponatraemia, hypokalaemia, hypophosphataemia, hypomagnesaemia, alkalosis), renal failure, sedative drugs (antipsychotics, benzodiazepines, opiates, antidepressants, barbiturates).

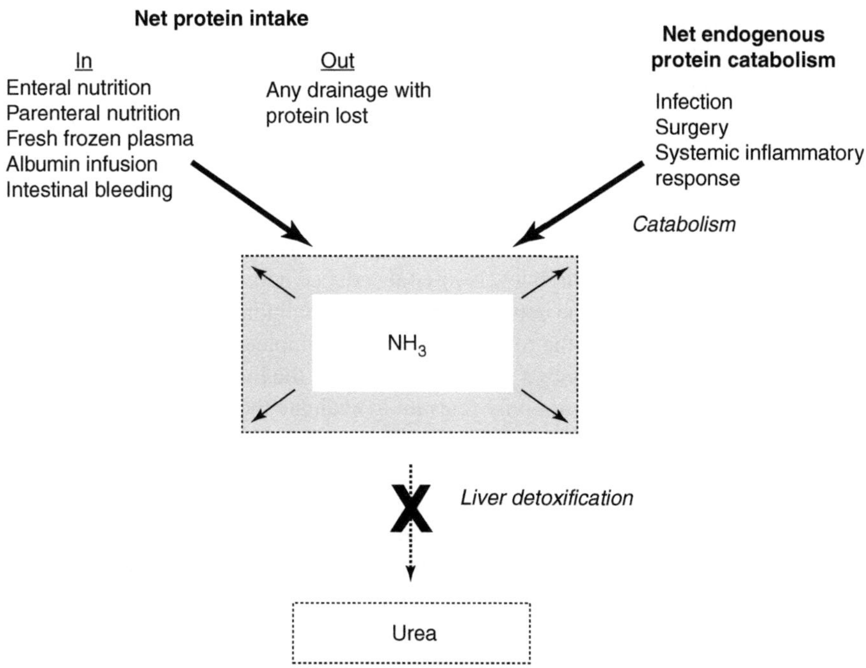

Fig. 1 Hyperammonaemia pathophysiology in acute liver failure. An increase in protein intake or protein catabolism is at risk to result in ammonia increase

Table 3 Differential diagnosis based on the results of standard laboratory tests for acute liver failure in newborns and infants

Test	Viral	Foetal alloimmune hepatitis	Indeterminate	Metabolic
ALT between	$8 - >20 \times N$	$N - <5 \times N$	$1.5–7 \times N$	$2–5 \times N$
GGT between	$2–3 \times N$	N	$N - 2 \times N$	$N–3 \times N$
Total bilirubin (mg/dL)	2–10	2–10	2–10	2–10
Direct bilirubin (mg/dL)	1–5	2–7	2–10	2–11
INR	2– >5	2– >5	2– >5	2–3

Laboratory Tests

Laboratory tests are important for diagnosis, to orient to the aetiology and to establish the severity of the liver injury. A summary of the diagnostic causes based on the results of standard laboratory tests for acute liver failure in newborns and infants are presented in Table 3.

Bilirubin levels are elevated in the majority of patients with acute liver failure. Normal or slightly elevated levels can orient to a metabolic disease (ex; tyrosinaemia), a drug ingestion with liver intoxication (ex; acetaminophen); or to a parvovirus-induced hepatic failure. In most patients a high increase of total bilirubin is observed, with a ratio between non-conjugated and conjugated bilirubin that is variable according to the degree of hepatocellular injury, being higher in patients with less remaining cells able to conjugate bilirubin or in those with associated haemolysis (e.g. Wilson disease).

The importance of the increase of *serum aminotransferase levels* can orient on the aetiological cause, being slightly elevated or normal in the foetal alloimmune hepatitis, could be of intermediate levels in diseases as autoimmune hepatitis and Wilson, and at high or very high levels in viral-induced hepatitis. Decrease of serum aminotransferase levels in the course of the disease can indicate either a decrease in the injury of the liver or be the result of its almost complete damage, mainly when this decrease is associated with a rapid diminution of the liver volume.

Glucose blood levels are not only relevant to evaluate the severity of the hepatocellular failure (hypoglycaemia), but they also could be low in metabolic diseases even with normal or mildly modified clotting factors.

Protein synthesis is also affected by the destruction of the hepatic parenchyma in metabolic diseases and toxic drugs/Xenobiotics, by viral infections or the inflammation generated by them. In cases of severe acute liver failure, clotting factors, proteins of short half-life (some hours), rapidly decrease in circulation, in contrast albumins having a half-life of around 3 weeks decrease lately in the course of the disease. High INR (International Normalized Ratio) or low percentage of PT (Prothrombin Time) indicate that the liver is not producing clotting factors. However, liver failure can frequently be complicated by bacterial infections and subsequently by disseminated intravascular coagulation that leads to consumption of circulating clotting factors, thus giving a false idea of the level of liver injury. The dosage of factor VIII is of help in such circumstances, because it is not produced by hepatocytes, thus not affected by the liver failure but reduced in cases of disseminated intravascular coagulation.

Blood urea nitrogen is produced in hepatocytes, thus serum levels are low in patients with liver failure. Serum creatinine level can be a better marker of renal function on those circumstances. *Ammonia* increase in serum is due to the failure of its transformation in blood urea nitrogen, levels are relatively well correlated with the degree of encephalopathy. Ammonia can be measured in venous or arterial blood samples that must be collected in a pre-chilled tube, transported in ice, and separated and analyzed immediately. Capillary samples should not be used, because of the presence of some haemolysis.

Complications

In acute liver failure, the massive destruction of hepatocytes is associated with many complications; its occurrence depends on the type of hepatocyte function affected by a particular aggressor or of the decrease of the liver mass (Fig. 2). Among the complications that may be encountered in fulminant hepatic failure, cerebral

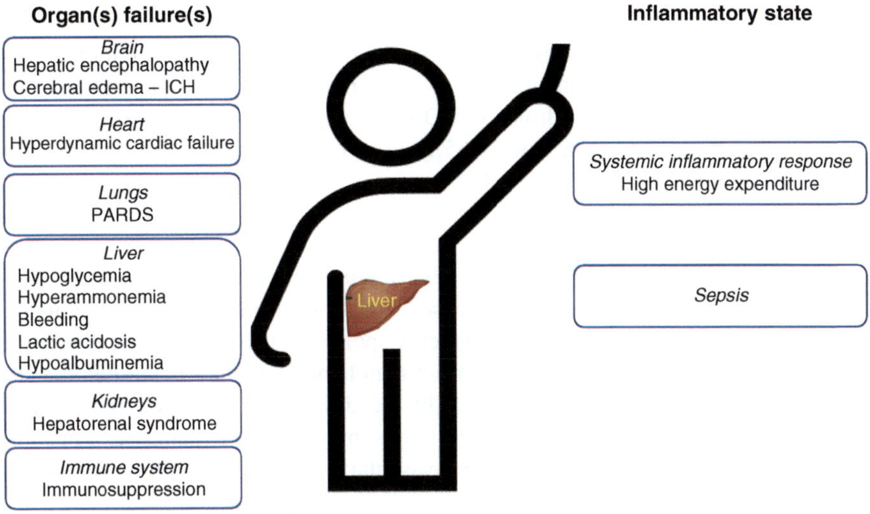

Fig. 2 Complications of acute liver failure. PARDS pediatric acute respiratory distress syndrome, ICH intracranial hypertension

oedema with brain hernia and multiple organ dysfunction syndromes are the two major leading causes of death. These complications are further detailed in specific book chapters.

In summary:

- *Cerebral oedema and intracranial hypertension*

Cerebral oedema complicates half of hepatic encephalopathies with coma (HE stage 3 or above). The pathophysiology is unclear and does not only involve increased ammonia levels but also other neurotoxics, osmotic stress, oxidative stress, inflammation mediators, and increased cerebral blood flow [62]. This cerebral oedema increases intracranial pressure that can lead to cerebral herniation and death, requiring an aggressive treatment when coma occurs, including extracorporeal treatment and emergency liver transplantation. In liver failure, the normal detoxification of ammonia to urea is impaired, and levels of circulating ammonia increase. There is a close relationship between an elevated ammonia level with the risk of intracranial hypertension leading to death, when there is a sustained level of ammonia ≥200 μmol per litre in children [63]. However, lower ammonia level can be associated with a severe encephalopathy.

- *Loss of vasomotor tone and hyperdynamic cardiac failure*

Vasodilation and elevated cardiac output with redistribution of blood flow to brain, skeletal muscles, and skin is frequently observed in severe liver failure. Clinically, a high cardiac index, normal filling pressures, and low systemic resistance are observed. The aetiology is poorly understood and may be due to the increase of inflammatory mediators normally cleared by the liver [64].

- *Acute respiratory failure*

Many complications may be responsible for respiratory failure in children with HE including aspiration, pneumonia, hypoventilation, and pleural effusion. An acute respiratory distress syndrome (ARDS), characterized by an hypoxaemia with new lung infiltrates on Chest X-Ray [65], can be observed in the most severe cases due to inflammation in the lungs [64].

- *Loss of liver metabolic functions*

Liver injury is responsible for hypoglycaemia, lactic acidosis, hypoalbuminaemia, and hyperammonaemia. The decrease in synthesis capacity of coagulation proteins can be responsible for haemorrhage. A spontaneous haemorrhagic syndrome affects less than 10% of patients with fulminant hepatic failure; most often the site of bleeding is the gastrointestinal tract. The bleeding is secondary to a reduction in clotting factors (all factors but factor VIII are synthetized by hepatocytes), in some cases to an associated disseminated intravascular coagulopathy with thrombocytopenia and increased fibrinolysis.

- *Renal failure and fluid overload*

Oliguric renal failure is associated with decreased survival. Interactive aetiologies include decrease intravascular volume due to water losses (urine losses due to mannitol osmotic diuresis), digestive losses (vomiting), third space (ascites), hypoalbuminaemia, sepsis and/or loss of vasomotor regulation. Usually serum urea blood level is of poor value, as urea production is low. According to the severity of the mechanism(s) involved, renal failure may correspond to prerenal azotemia, acute tubular necrosis or hepato-renal syndrome.

- *Sepsis and impaired immune response*

Sepsis and impaired immune response are common in acute liver failure, due to decrease in liver clearance of translocate enteric organisms. It is sometimes difficult to differentiate sepsis from loss of vasomotor tone due to liver failure.

All this complications can be associated with different severity levels and are regrouped in the terminology “multiple organ dysfunction syndrome”. The quantification of the severity the multiple organ failure syndrome can be done using the PELOD 2 score [66].

Treatments

The severity of illness, rapidity of clinical changes, and the potential needs of a liver transplantation require early critical care management with non-specific and specific treatments.

Non-specific Treatments

Acute liver failure must be considered as a life-threatening condition. A symptomatic treatment is urgently indicated including intravascular bolus associated or not to norepinephrine in case of shock; intubation, nasogastric tube, and mannitol infusion (0.5 g/kg mannitol 20%) in case of coma; phenytoin if seizures; and infusion of 0.5–1 g/kg/h of dextrose 10–20% with a rapid insertion of a central line, in case of hypoglycaemia. After stabilization, the child should be rapidly referred to a paediatric intensive care unit in a hospital with a liver transplantation program.

> After stabilization, a child with acute liver failure should be rapidly referred to a paediatric intensive care unit in a hospital with a liver transplantation program.

The management depends on the organ failure severity:

Respiratory management:

Mechanical ventilation with airway protection is indicated if Glasgow coma score is below 8 (HE stage 2–3). Sedation should be as minimal as possible to appropriately assess neurologic status. Ventilator support is set to maintain an oxygen saturation above 95% and a close to normal $PaCO_2$ and pH, to limit increase of cerebral blood flow due to acidosis, and diffusion of ammonia across the blood brain barrier in case of alkalosis.

- *Haemodynamic management:*

The increase in intracranial pressure and the frequent loss of cerebral autoregulation requires maintaining plasma volume and blood pressure. The first step is to infuse saline 0.9% bolus (avoid Ringer lactate), if necessary start an infusion of norepinephrine. Cerebral perfusion is followed with transcranial Doppler. Low doses of hydrocortisone can help to reduce norepinephrine posology [67].

- *Neurologic management*

Prevention of HE aggravating factors (see above) is the baseline of the treatment in patients with acute liver failure. An active treatment of intracranial hypertension (ICH) is usually performed in children with HE stage ≥3. These children are mechanically ventilated with the lower possible sedation. Mannitol infusion of 0.5 g/kg/dose is performed with osmolality monitoring [68] eventually replaced after 3–4 doses by Saline 3% to maintain osmolality between 310 and 330 mOsm/L and serum sodium level between 145 and 150 mmol/L. A body core temperature of 36–37 °C is maintained as a moderate hypothermia did not show any benefit [69, 70]. To refine the ICH treatments, intracranial pressure is rarely monitored as it requires an invasive intracranial probe with high bleeding risk. Indirect assessment of cerebral blood oxygenation with near infrared spectroscopy and intermittent assessment of cerebral blood perfusion with transcranial Doppler, help pediatric intensivists to assess treatment effects and ICH evolution.

Hyperammoniaemia is an important cause of HE;, therefore, its prevention and treatment must be a priority of the management (Fig. 2). The initial approach consists in the decrease of proteins or amino acids intake or administration, administration of lactulose, a non-absorbable carbohydrate acting as an osmotic laxative, and orally non-absorbable antibiotics to decrease bacteria concentration in the colon. In the absence of inborn error of metabolism, the benefit of a treatment of hyperammonaemia with sodium benzoate and sodium phenylbutyrate is not demonstrated but can be initiated to control hyperammonaemia before an extracorporeal removal therapy is considered.

- *Water balance and metabolic management*

Water and sodium restriction, in the absence of ICH, helps to control water and sodium balance in those children who usually have secondary hyperaldosteronism. Albumin infusion (1 g/kg) is indicated to maintain oncotic pressure according to albumin blood level.

- *Hematological management*

Systematic infusion of fresh frozen plasma (FFP) to correct INR is not recommended as it can be responsible for water overload and increase protein intake with augmented ammonia blood level. After FFP infusion, INR or factor V does not correlate with liver synthesis function for 8–12 h, interfering with the interpretation of the degree of liver failure, thus with the indication of a liver transplant. FFP is reserved to three situations: (1) active bleeding, (2) any invasive procedure, (3) preparation for liver transplantation. In case of intractable bleeding, *recombinant factor VIIa can help to control the bleeding. To limit fluid overload, therapeutic plasma exchange can be used to administer FFP (see below).*

Platelet transfusion is indicated if active bleeding or platelet count is below $30–50.10^9$/L

- *Nutritional support*

Enteral nutrition is maintained as long as possible. The diet includes low protein (0.5 g/kg/24 h), high carbohydrate, low sodium with normal vitamin and trace elements intakes. In case of hypoglycaemia severe hepatocyte function impairment, a continuous intravenous glucose infusion is maintained to avoid any recurrent hypoglycaemia episode.

- *Other support*

Drugs dose is adjusted to liver metabolism decrease. Antibiotics are started as soon as infection is suspected.

Specific Treatments

The aetiological diagnosis of the acute liver failure is of paramount importance in all age groups, because of the availability of specific treatments for some causes of severe acute liver injury. In addition, in diagnosis of malignant liver infiltration, a liver transplant is usually contraindicated.

In newborns with acute liver failure, in the absence of initial diagnosis, galactose is removed from the diet and acyclovir is started until both galactosaemia and herpes virus infection are excluded as responsible for the liver damage. Galactoasemia and fructosaemia need a diet without any galactose or fructose. Viral infection can be treated with specific antiviral drug; as example, intravenous administration of acyclovir for HSV, ganciclovir for CMV, or cidofovir for adenovirus infections [71].

In newborns with foetal alloimmune hepatitis, exchange transfusion and intravenous immunoglobulins improve outcome, reducing also the need for a liver transplantation [32]. The diagnosis of this disorder is relevant to deliver the correct treatment, but also to set up a preventive treatment in future pregnancies. In case of antecedents of foetal alloimmune hepatitis, maternal treatment with antenatal intravenous Ig infusions (1 g/kg weekly of immunoglobulins from the week 18th of gestation) avoids the development of severe liver failure. Newborns from treated mothers show no or only mild signs of transient hepatitis [31].

N'Acetyl-cysteine is the treatment of patients with acetaminophen-induced acute liver failure, providing cysteine as a substrate for glutathione synthesis [72]. In addition, N'Acetyl-cysteine could also form adducts with the toxic metabolite of acetaminophen (N-acetyl-p-benzoquinoneimine), improve haemodynamics and oxygen use, and decrease cerebral oedema [73]. This agent shows low toxicity, very good tolerance, explaining why it is used in patients with acetaminophen overdose even if they do not have hepatic failure or are not at risk according to the ingested dose. The risk of patients with repeated ingestion of large doses cannot be stratified using the Rumack-Matthew normogram; in these individuals use of N-Acetyl-Cysteine is more liberal, some authors recommend starting immediately when serum levels of acetaminophen are higher than 20 μg/ml [73]. Intravenous dose of 150 mg/kg, administered in 15–60 min, followed by 12.5 mg/kg/h over 4 h, and then by 6.25 mg/kg/h over 16 h, are recommended by the FDA. Oral administration, in case that this is the pathway of choice, consists in a loading dose of 140 mg/kg, followed by 17 doses of 70 mg/kg repeated every 4 h (FDA protocol). No data is available indicating the superiority of one or another administration modality. However, the medication has an unpleasant smell and taste, and vomiting is a usual symptom when administered orally. Around 5% of treated patients can show adverse effects, being the urticarial and even anaphylactic reactions the most frequent ones. No measurable acetaminophen concentration is a good parameter to decide stopping the treatment. These protocols, mainly the intravenous one, can be short and the choice to carry on or stop the infusion should be the responsibility of the caring physician according to clinical and laboratory features.

N'Acetyl-Cysteine has been proposed in non-acetaminophen-induced hepatic failure; however, it does not improve transplantation free-survival, thus those results do not support its use out of the context of acetaminophen-induced liver injury [74].

Immunosuppressive drugs should be administered to infants or children with Giant cell hepatitis associated with a Coombs positive haemolytic anaemia. Rituximab (anti-CD20 antibodies) could be used at onset, but associated with another drug, because plasmocytes survive to Rituximab for 3 or 4 weeks since they do not express CD20.

Administration of immunosuppressive drugs, mainly corticosteroids, in patients with fulminant form of autoimmune, is controversial. No clinical, biochemical, or histological marker predicts the treatment outcome. The use of these drugs must be balanced with the potential consequences if the patient requires a liver transplant, as the increase (risk of post-transplant infections).

In patients with Wilson disease, initiation of a Cu++ chelator therapy (D-Penicillamine) could be indicated; however, it should be considered that these therapies need relatively long time to be effective. Recently, tetrathiomolybdate has been shown to be effective; however, prospective studies on its toxicity are still tested [75].

Benzylpenicillin (Penicillin G) and ceftazidime are B-lactam antibiotics thought to be hepatoprotective in amatoxin poisoning. Association of the B -lactam with Silymarin is a very efficient therapy for amanita intoxication. The value of sylimarin relates to the lag between ingest of mushrooms and administration of the medication. When the drug is administered in the first 48 h, it prevents severe liver injury. Side effects are nausea, epigastric discomfort, arthralgia, headaches, pruritus, and urticarial, has been reported [76]. Initial dose of silybin dihemisuccinate is 5 mg/kg by IV infusion over 1 h followed by 20 mg/kg/day by continuous infusion for 6 days until transaminase levels have normalized. No research is available to support its use in children under 12 years of age, thus it is not administered unless the benefits outweigh the risks [77].

Specific diet with low Tyrosine, Phenylalanine and Methionine and Nitisinone (NTBC) improve liver failure in patients with tyrosinaemia, without need for an emergency liver transplant.

Extracorporeal Therapy as a Bridge to Liver Transplantation

Orthotopic liver transplantation remains the only effective treatment in many children with acute liver failure. When children have a hepatic encephalopathy stage ≥3, high volume haemofiltration defined as an ultrafiltrate flow ≥80 ml/kg/h is the first choice to mitigate brain damage while waiting for a liver transplant. Molecular absorbent Recirculating System (MARS®: Gambro, Lund Sweden) can also be used in children above 1 year old, in combination with high volume haemofiltration. Some authors propose to therapeutic plasma exchange in combination with the previous treatment in order to treat the coagulopathy without increasing fluid overload (see chapter Liver Failure and Extracorporeal Therapies) [78, 79]. However, randomized clinical trials are still needed to define the best extracorporeal treatment [80].

Prognosis

An important concern in clinical practice is the prediction of the outcome in patients with acute liver failure. The most relevant decision is to establish who needs a liver transplant. No available score system accurately predicts death without liver transplantation. Reasons to explain difficulties in proposing an ideal model are mainly the high diversity of liver diseases presenting as an acute liver failure in children, and also the variation of aetiologies at different ages. A score system has been proposed for patients with Wilson disease [81], showing good sensitivity and specificity of 88% and 90%, respectively. However, application to a different cohort of patients was not accurate [54]. In particular aetiologies, such as Wilson disease, prognosis varies according to the presence or absence of encephalopathy in between 81.5% and 32.4%, respectively.

However, several studies showed that Liver Injury Units (LIU) score, PELD, or even King's College scores can be used in particular circumstances. The variety of aetiologies of acute liver failure in children with their own natural history and possible therapeutic options complicate the use of a unique score in all cases. Currently, around 45% of children with an acute liver failure are transplanted [82].

The LIU score was calculated using the peak laboratory values of total bilirubin, blood ammonia, prothrombine time, or INR. In a multicentre cohort, this score was found to be a good predictor of transplant-free survival, but it was less useful to predict death without liver transplantation. This score was not helpful when LIU was calculated using data at the admission. In addition, LIU is less predictive in children under the age of 6 months [82].

King's College criteria showed a high sensitivity and specificity, as well as positive and negative predictive values when applied to a population of children in which the main causes of acute liver failure were HAV, and indeterminate hepatitis. Such analysis was made including or excluding liver-transplanted patients [83]. Different results were reported in another study in which the primary outcome was survival without liver transplantation vs. death at 21 days following enrolment. Data showed a very low positive predictive value (33%) and a high negative predictive value of 88% using the King's College score. Interestingly, in that cohort of 215 children with acute liver failure, a multivariate analysis for end-point mortality identified as independents predictors: the peak of bilirubin, PT/INR levels, and hepatic encephalopathy. This study also showed that survival varies between frequent aetiologies, from more than 30% in Hepatitis A Virus (HAV) to 16% in indeterminate cases. This was also the case in between types of onset, being 24% in hyperacute cases, 27% in acute onset, and 6.7% in subacute liver failure. Applying a different classification, similar results are found, showing that survival is less frequent in patients with a subfulminant form of liver failure [83].

PELD (Paediatric End-stage Liver Disease) score, initially described for establishment of priority for children in the waiting list for a liver transplant, was tested on children in hepatic failure with good results for establishing the time for liver transplantation. The cut-off was established at 33, being higher at admission for non-survivors and recipients of a liver transplant [84]. In addition, PELD score, and King's College score were similarly predictive of outcome.

The level of inflammation markers could help in establishing a prognosis.

Continuous evaluation is necessary to decide the inclusion of children in the liver transplantation waiting list.

Conclusions

Paediatric acute liver failure is a severe complication of metabolic, viral, toxic, and autoimmune injuries. In newborns and infants, metabolic causes are the most frequently found. In many of these cases, no indication for a liver transplantation exists; because specific treatments have been developed for some of them or by the presence of extra-hepatic diseases that cannot be cured by a liver transplant.

Currently, in children of more than 1 year of age, indeterminate hepatitis is the main diagnosis, in some cases complicated by bone marrow aplasia. Leucopenia, thrombocytopenia, and anaemia can present after a liver transplantation. To decrease the number of patients classified as having an indeterminate hepatitis, testing for all possible causative viruses, as well as autoimmune liver diseases, and serum levels of acetaminophen should be rapidly done.

Specific treatments exist for many causes of acute liver failure that when applied early show a high percentage of success. Extensive testing for those aetiologies must be done according to clinical, laboratory, and radiologic results. Toxicity should always be suspected, and rigorous questioning of patients and parents required. Measures tending to prevent usual complications are indicated. Preventive or replacement treatments must be carefully evaluated and carried out in a centre with a program of liver transplantation. Encephalopathy is of difficult diagnosis in young children; sometimes the only sign could be a subtle change in the child behaviour. However, even in absence of clinical signs of encephalopathy, serum ammonia levels should be maintained as low as possible. Extra-corporeal support systems have not been carefully and rigorously evaluated in children, thus its indication is not recommended in the absence of a life-threatening condition (see above).

No prognostic models have been designed for paediatric acute liver failure, since causes are different according to the patient age, and for many of them a treatment is possible, development of a score system becomes difficult. For older children with indeterminate hepatitis or Wilson disease, score systems set up by adults and paediatric hepatologists at the King's College could be applied.

References

1. Squires RH Jr, Shneider BL, Bucuvalas J, Alonso E, Sokol RJ, Narkewicz MR, et al. Acute liver failure in children: the first 348 patients in the pediatric acute liver failure study group. J Pediatr. 2006;148(5):652–8.
2. O'Grady JG, Schalm SW, Williams R. Acute liver failure: redefining the syndromes. Lancet. 1993;342(8866):273–5.
3. Sundaram SS, Alonso EM, Narkewicz MR, Zhang S, Squires RH. Characterization and outcomes of young infants with acute liver failure. J Pediatr. 2011;159(5):813–8.
4. Taylor SA, Whitington PF. Neonatal acute liver failure. Liver Transpl. 2016;22(5):677–85.
5. Durand P, Debray D, Mandel R, Baujard C, Branchereau S, Gauthier F, et al. Acute liver failure in infancy: a 14-year experience of a pediatric liver transplantation center. J Pediatr. 2001;139(6):871–6.
6. Dhawan A. Etiology and prognosis of acute liver failure in children. Liver Transpl. 2008;14(Suppl 2):S80–4.
7. Shanmugam NP, Bansal S, Greenough A, Verma A, Dhawan A. Neonatal liver failure: aetiologies and management--state of the art. Eur J Pediatr. 2011;170(5):573–81.
8. Saudubray JM, Nassogne MC, de Lonlay P, Touati G. Clinical approach to inherited metabolic disorders in neonates: an overview. Semin Neonatol. 2002;7(1):3–15.
9. Mitchell GRP, Dubois J, Alvarez F. Tyrosinemia. Liver disease in children. New York: Cambridge, University Press; 2014. p. 694–713.
10. Li H, Byers HM, Diaz-Kuan A, Vos MB, Hall PL, Tortorelli S, et al. Acute liver failure in neonates with undiagnosed hereditary fructose intolerance due to exposure from widely available infant formulas. Mol Genet Metab. 2018;123(4):428–32.
11. Kisler JE, Whittaker RG, McFarland R. Mitochondrial diseases in childhood: a clinical approach to investigation and management. Dev Med Child Neurol. 2010;52(5):422–33.
12. Schapira AH. Mitochondrial diseases. Lancet. 2012;379(9828):1825–34.
13. Schon EA, DiMauro S, Hirano M. Human mitochondrial DNA: roles of inherited and somatic mutations. Nat Rev Genet. 2012;13(12):878–90.
14. Lightowlers RN, Taylor RW, Turnbull DM. Mutations causing mitochondrial disease: what is new and what challenges remain? Science. 2015;349(6255):1494–9.
15. Gaignard P, Gonzales E, Ackermann O, Labrune P, Correia I, Therond P, et al. Mitochondrial infantile liver disease due to TRMU gene mutations: three new cases. JIMD Rep. 2013;11:117–23.
16. Lenz D, McClean P, Kansu A, Bonnen PE, Ranucci G, Thiel C, et al. SCYL1 variants cause a syndrome with low gamma-glutamyl-transferase cholestasis, acute liver failure, and neurodegeneration (CALFAN). Genet Med. 2018;20(10):1255–65.
17. Haack TB, Staufner C, Kopke MG, Straub BK, Kolker S, Thiel C, et al. Biallelic mutations in NBAS cause recurrent acute liver failure with onset in infancy. Am J Hum Genet. 2015;97(1):163–9.
18. Houten SM, Wanders RJ. A general introduction to the biochemistry of mitochondrial fatty acid beta-oxidation. J Inherit Metab Dis. 2010;33(5):469–77.
19. Olivier F, Wieckowska A, Piedboeuf B, Alvarez F. Cholestasis and hepatic failure in a neonate: a case report of severe pyruvate kinase deficiency. Pediatrics. 2015;136(5):e1366–8.

20. Chartier ME, Hart L, Paganelli M, Ahmed N, Bilodeau M, Alvarez F. Successful liver transplants for liver failure associated with pyruvate kinase deficiency. Pediatrics. 2018;141(Suppl 5):S385–S9.
21. Batshaw ML, Tuchman M, Summar M, Seminara J. Members of the urea cycle disorders C. A longitudinal study of urea cycle disorders. Mol Genet Metab. 2014;113(1–2):127–30.
22. Braissant O. Current concepts in the pathogenesis of urea cycle disorders. Mol Genet Metab. 2010;100(Suppl 1):S3–S12.
23. Schwarz KB, Dell Olio D, Lobritto SJ, Lopez MJ, Rodriguez-Baez N, Yazigi NA, et al. Analysis of viral testing in nonacetaminophen pediatric acute liver failure. J Pediatr Gastroenterol Nutr. 2014;59(5):616–23.
24. Narkewicz MR, Horslen S, Hardison RM, Shneider BL, Rodriguez-Baez N, Alonso EM, et al. A learning collaborative approach increases specificity of diagnosis of acute liver failure in pediatric patients. Clin Gastroenterol Hepatol. 2018;16(11):1801–10 e3.
25. Dupuy JM, Frommel D, Alagille D. Severe viral hepatitis type B in infancy. Lancet. 1975;1(7900):191–4.
26. Zhang K, Chandrakasan S, Chapman H, Valencia CA, Husami A, Kissell D, et al. Synergistic defects of different molecules in the cytotoxic pathway lead to clinical familial hemophagocytic lymphohistiocytosis. Blood. 2014;124(8):1331–4.
27. Wegehaupt O, Wustrau K, Lehmberg K, Ehl S. Cell versus cytokine - directed therapies for Hemophagocytic Lymphohistiocytosis (HLH) in inborn errors of immunity. Front Immunol. 2020;11:808.
28. Whitington PF, Pan X, Kelly S, Melin-Aldana H, Malladi P. Gestational alloimmune liver disease in cases of fetal death. J Pediatr. 2011;159(4):612–6.
29. Debray FG, de Halleux V, Guidi O, Detrembleur N, Gaillez S, Rausin L, et al. Neonatal liver cirrhosis without iron overload caused by gestational alloimmune liver disease. Pediatrics. 2012;129(4):e1076–e9.
30. Bonilla S, Prozialeck JD, Malladi P, Pan X, Yu S, Melin-Aldana H, et al. Neonatal iron overload and tissue siderosis due to gestational alloimmune liver disease. J Hepatol. 2012;56(6):1351–5.
31. Baruteau J, Heissat S, Broue P, Collardeau-Frachon S, Bouvier R, Fabre M, et al. Transient neonatal liver disease after maternal antenatal intravenous Ig infusions in gestational alloimmune liver disease associated with neonatal haemochromatosis. J Pediatr Gastroenterol Nutr. 2014;59(5):629–35.
32. Rand EB, Karpen SJ, Kelly S, Mack CL, Malatack JJ, Sokol RJ, et al. Treatment of neonatal hemochromatosis with exchange transfusion and intravenous immunoglobulin. J Pediatr. 2009;155(4):566–71.
33. Bernard O, Hadchouel M, Scotto J, Odievre M, Alagille D. Severe giant cell hepatitis with autoimmune hemolytic anemia in early childhood. J Pediatr. 1981;99(5):704–11.
34. Maggiore G, Sciveres M, Fabre M, Gori L, Pacifico L, Resti M, et al. Giant cell hepatitis with autoimmune hemolytic anemia in early childhood: long-term outcome in 16 children. J Pediatr. 2011;159(1):127–32.
35. Paganelli M, Patey N, Bass LM, Alvarez F. Anti-CD20 treatment of giant cell hepatitis with autoimmune hemolytic anemia. Pediatrics. 2014;134(4):e1206–10.
36. Grzywacz K, Brochu P, Beaunoyer M, Lallier M, Alvarez F. Neonatal peliosis with maternal ingestion of pesticides. J Pediatr Gastroenterol Nutr. 2014;58(2):e14–e7.
37. Maggiore G, Socie G, Sciveres M, Roque-Afonso AM, Nastasio S, Johanet C, et al. Seronegative autoimmune hepatitis in children: spectrum of disorders. Dig Liver Dis. 2016;48(7):785–91.
38. Alonso EM, Horslen SP, Behrens EM, Doo E. Pediatric acute liver failure of undetermined cause: a research workshop. Hepatology. 2017;65(3):1026–37.
39. Chapin CA, Melin-Aldana H, Kreiger PA, Burn T, Neighbors K, Taylor SA, et al. Activated CD8 T-cell hepatitis in children with indeterminate acute liver failure: results from a multicenter cohort. J Pediatr Gastroenterol Nutr. 2020;71(6):713–9.
40. Sokal EM, Melchior M, Cornu C, Vandenbroucke AT, Buts JP, Cohen BJ, et al. Acute parvovirus B19 infection associated with fulminant hepatitis of favourable prognosis in young children. Lancet. 1998;352(9142):1739–41.

41. Bathla L, Grant WJ, Mercer DF, Vargas LM, Gebhart CL, Langnas AN. Parvovirus associated fulminant hepatic failure and aplastic anemia treated successfully with liver and bone marrow transplantation. A report of two cases. Am J Transplant. 2014;14(11):2645–50.
42. Uetrecht J, Kaplowitz N. Inhibition of immune tolerance unmasks drug-induced allergic hepatitis. Hepatology. 2015;62(2):346–8.
43. Alonso EM, James LP, Zhang S, Squires RH. Acetaminophen adducts detected in serum of Pediatric patients with acute liver failure. J Pediatr Gastroenterol Nutr. 2015;61(1):102–7.
44. Shah AD, Wood DM, Dargan PI. Understanding lactic acidosis in paracetamol (acetaminophen) poisoning. Br J Clin Pharmacol. 2011;71(1):20–8.
45. Shi Q, Yang X, Greenhaw JJ, Salminen AT, Russotti GM, Salminen WF. Drug-induced liver injury in children: clinical observations, animal models, and regulatory status. Int J Toxicol. 2017;36(5):365–79.
46. Li S, Guo J, Ying Z, Chen S, Yang L, Chen K, et al. Valproic acid-induced hepatotoxicity in Alpers syndrome is associated with mitochondrial permeability transition pore opening-dependent apoptotic sensitivity in an induced pluripotent stem cell model. Hepatology. 2015;61(5):1730–9.
47. Klein AS, Hart J, Brems JJ, Goldstein L, Lewin K, Busuttil RW. Amanita poisoning: treatment and the role of liver transplantation. Am J Med. 1989;86(2):187–93.
48. Maggiore G, Porta G, Bernard O, Hadchouel M, Alvarez F, Homberg JC, et al. Autoimmune hepatitis with initial presentation as acute hepatic failure in young children. J Pediatr. 1990;116(2):280–2.
49. Porta G, Gayotto LC, Alvarez F. Anti-liver-kidney microsome antibody-positive autoimmune hepatitis presenting as fulminant liver failure. J Pediatr Gastroenterol Nutr. 1990;11(1):138–40.
50. Herzog D, Rasquin-Weber AM, Debray D, Alvarez F. Subfulminant hepatic failure in autoimmune hepatitis type 1: an unusual form of presentation. J Hepatol. 1997;27(3):578–82.
51. Cuarterolo ML, Ciocca ME, Lopez SI, de Davila MT, Alvarez F. Immunosuppressive therapy allows recovery from liver failure in children with autoimmune hepatitis. Clin Gastroenterol Hepatol. 2011;9(2):145–9.
52. Hayashi H, Tatsumi Y, Yahata S, Hayashi H, Momose K, Isaji R, et al. Acute hepatic phenotype of Wilson disease: clinical features of acute episodes and chronic lesions remaining in survivors. J Clin Transl Hepatol. 2015;3(4):239–45.
53. Ohya Y, Okajima H, Honda M, Hayashida S, Suda H, Matsumoto S, et al. Re-evaluation of the indications for liver transplantation in Wilson's disease based on the outcomes of patients referred to a transplant center. Pediatr Transplant. 2013;17(4):369–73.
54. Fischer RT, Soltys KA, Squires RH Jr, Jaffe R, Mazariegos GV, Shneider BL. Prognostic scoring indices in Wilson disease: a case series and cautionary tale. J Pediatr Gastroenterol Nutr. 2011;52(4):466–9.
55. Rivet C, Leverger G, Jacquemin E, Bernard O. Acute leukemia presenting as acute hepatitis without liver failure. J Pediatr Gastroenterol Nutr. 2014;59(5):640–1.
56. Takahashi H, Sakai R, Hattori Y, Ohshima R, Kuwabara H, Hagihara M, et al. Successful disease control with L-asparaginase monotherapy for aggressive natural killer cell leukemia with severe hepatic failure. Leuk Lymphoma. 2013;54(3):662–4.
57. Zafrani ES, Gaulard P. Primary lymphoma of the liver. Liver. 1993;13(2):57–61.
58. Rowbotham D, Wendon J, Williams R. Acute liver failure secondary to hepatic infiltration: a single centre experience of 18 cases. Gut. 1998;42(4):576–80.
59. Lettieri CJ, Berg BW. Clinical features of non-Hodgkins lymphoma presenting with acute liver failure: a report of five cases and review of published experience. Am J Gastroenterol. 2003;98(7):1641–6.
60. Visnyei K, Grossbard ML, Shapira I. Hepatosplenic gammadelta T-cell lymphoma: an overview. Clin Lymphoma Myeloma Leuk. 2013;13(4):360–9.
61. Roscioli T, Cliffe ST, Bloch DB, Bell CG, Mullan G, Taylor PJ, et al. Mutations in the gene encoding the PML nuclear body protein Sp110 are associated with immunodeficiency and hepatic veno-occlusive disease. Nat Genet. 2006;38(6):620–2.

62. Ducharme-Crevier LD-TG, Lortie A, Maranda B, Tasker RC, Jouvet P. Metabolic encephalopathies in children. In: Lippincott WW, editor. Nichols DG Rogers textbook of pediatric intensive care. 5th ed. Philadelphia: Wolters Kluwer; 2016. p. 1053–65.
63. Ozanne B, Nelson J, Cousineau J, Lambert M, Phan V, Mitchell G, et al. Threshold for toxicity from hyperammonemia in critically ill children. J Hepatol. 2012;56(1):123–8.
64. Bernal W, Wendon J. Acute liver failure. N Engl J Med. 2013;369(26):2525–34.
65. Group PALICC. Pediatric acute respiratory distress syndrome: consensus recommendations from the Pediatric acute lung injury consensus conference. Pediatr Crit Care Med. 2015;16(5):428–39.
66. Leteurtre S, Duhamel A, Salleron J, Grandbastien B, Lacroix J, Leclerc F, et al. PELOD-2: an update of the PEdiatric logistic organ dysfunction score. Crit Care Med. 2013;41(7):1761–73.
67. Harry R, Auzinger G, Wendon J. The effects of supraphysiological doses of corticosteroids in hypotensive liver failure. Liver Int. 2003;23(2):71–7.
68. Jalan R. Intracranial hypertension in acute liver failure: pathophysiological basis of rational management. Semin Liver Dis. 2003;23(3):271–82.
69. Jalan R, Olde Damink SW, Deutz NE, Hayes PC, Lee A. Moderate hypothermia in patients with acute liver failure and uncontrolled intracranial hypertension. Gastroenterology. 2004;127(5):1338–46.
70. Bitzer M, Horger M, Giannini EG, Ganten TM, Worns MA, Siveke JT, et al. Resminostat plus sorafenib as second-line therapy of advanced hepatocellular carcinoma - the SHELTER study. J Hepatol. 2016;65(2):280–8.
71. Ganapathi L, Arnold A, Jones S, Patterson A, Graham D, Harper M, et al. Use of cidofovir in pediatric patients with adenovirus infection. F1000Res. 2016;5:758.
72. Lee WM, Hynan LS, Rossaro L, Fontana RJ, Stravitz RT, Larson AM, et al. Intravenous N-acetylcysteine improves transplant-free survival in early stage non-acetaminophen acute liver failure. Gastroenterology. 2009;137(3):856–64.
73. Heard KJ. Acetylcysteine for acetaminophen poisoning. N Engl J Med. 2008;359(3):285–92.
74. Squires RH, Dhawan A, Alonso E, Narkewicz MR, Shneider BL, Rodriguez-Baez N, et al. Intravenous N-acetylcysteine in pediatric patients with nonacetaminophen acute liver failure: a placebo-controlled clinical trial. Hepatology. 2013;57(4):1542–9.
75. Weiss KH, Askari FK, Czlonkowska A, Ferenci P, Bronstein JM, Bega D, et al. Bis-choline tetrathiomolybdate in patients with Wilson's disease: an open-label, multicentre, phase 2 study. Lancet Gastroenterol Hepatol. 2017;2(12):869–76.
76. Enjalbert F, Rapior S, Nouguier-Soule J, Guillon S, Amouroux N, Cabot C. Treatment of amatoxin poisoning: 20-year retrospective analysis. J Toxicol Clin Toxicol. 2002;40(6):715–57.
77. Wellington K, Jarvis B. Silymarin: a review of its clinical properties in the management of hepatic disorders. BioDrugs. 2001;15(7):465–89.
78. Larsen FS, Schmidt LE, Bernsmeier C, Rasmussen A, Isoniemi H, Patel VC, et al. High-volume plasma exchange in patients with acute liver failure: an open randomised controlled trial. J Hepatol. 2016;64(1):69–78.
79. Schaefer B, Schaefer F, Engelmann G, Meyburg J, Heckert KH, Zorn M, et al. Comparison of molecular adsorbents recirculating system (MARS) dialysis with combined plasma exchange and haemodialysis in children with acute liver failure. Nephrol Dial Transplant. 2011;26(11):3633–9.
80. Merouani A, Jouvet P. High-volume hemofiltration for critically ill children with acute liver failure: a standard treatment? Pediatr Crit Care Med. 2014;15(7):681–3.
81. Dhawan A, Taylor RM, Cheeseman P, De SP, Katsiyiannakis L, Mieli-Vergani G. Wilson's disease in children: 37-year experience and revised King's score for liver transplantation. Liver Transpl. 2005;11(4):441–8.
82. Lu BR, Zhang S, Narkewicz MR, Belle SH, Squires RH, Sokol RJ. Evaluation of the liver injury unit scoring system to predict survival in a multinational study of pediatric acute liver failure. J Pediatr. 2013;162(5):1010–6.
83. Ciocca M, Ramonet M, Cuarterolo M, Lopez S, Cernadas C, Alvarez F. Prognostic factors in paediatric acute liver failure. Arch Dis Child. 2008;93(1):48–51.
84. Sanchez MC, D'Agostino DE. Pediatric end-stage liver disease score in acute liver failure to assess poor prognosis. J Pediatr Gastroenterol Nutr. 2012;54(2):193–6.

Acute-on-Chronic Liver Failure

Marie-Eve Chartier and Fernando Alvarez

Acute-on-chronic liver failure (ACLF) must be considered when acute decompensation, resulting from various insults, is associated with rapid deterioration of hepatic function or extrahepatic organ failure. This new concept is different from the standard acute decompensation of cirrhosis and is associated with high short-term mortality, similar to patients with acute liver failure and considerably higher than anticipated with decompensated cirrhosis [1]. This syndrome can occur in patients having until then compensated cirrhosis or can represent the first manifestation of the liver disease, being frequently more severe in the former patients. The incidence and prevalence of this syndrome in children is unknown, but in adults, it represents around 20–30% of admissions in cirrhotic patients. Given the high mortality rate associated with ACLF, compared to acute decompensation of cirrhosis, it is important to recognize early patients with ACLF, as organ allocation, timing of transplant and prognostication will be influenced.

Definitions and Diagnostic Criteria

Over the last two decades, ACLF has been proposed as a distinctive condition from decompensated cirrhosis. However, more than a decade ago, there was no consistent definition of ACLF in the literature and each study used its own definition. In 2009, the Asian Pacific Association for the Study of the Liver (APASL) [2]

M.-E. Chartier (✉)
Division of Gastroenterology, Hepatology and Nutrition, CHU Sainte-Justine, Université de Montréal, Montreal, QC, Canada
e-mail: marie-eve.chartier@mail.mcgill.ca

F. Alvarez
Division of Gastroenterology, Hepatology & Nutrition, Department of Pediatrics of Sainte Justine Hospital, University of Montreal, Montréal, QC, Canada
e-mail: fernando.alvarez@umontreal.ca

P. Jouvet, F. Alvarez (eds.), *Liver Diseases in the Pediatric Intensive Care Unit*,
https://doi.org/10.1007/978-3-030-79132-2_3

Table 1 Modified pediatric acute-on-chronic liver failure definition: P-CLIF

Diagnosis	All patients with chronic liver disease. Exclusion of malignancies and some metabolic disorders: urea cycle and maple syrup urine disease
Severity marker	Change in calculated MELD/PELD of ≥10 in 28–90 days PLUS two of the following (one if renal failure)
Jaundice	Bilirubin ≥205 μmol/L
Coagulopathy	INR >2.5
Renal dysfunction/failure	*Dysfunction:* Infant: serum Cr > 44 μmol/L Child (1–12 y.o): serum Cr > 80 μmol/L Adolescent (12–18 y.o): serum Cr > 115 μmol/L *Failure:* Renal replacement therapy OR Infant: serum Cr > 62 μmol/L Child: serum Cr > 106 μmol/L Adolescent: serum Cr > 141 μmol/L
Cerebral dysfunction/failure	*Dysfunction:* Grade I or II hepatic encephalopathy *Failure:* Grade III or IV hepatic encephalopathy
Respiratory failure	Mechanical ventilation
Circulatory failure	Use of inotropes/pressors

suggested the first accepted criteria based on expert consensus from single center studies. Recently, the definition has been modernized according to two large prospective studies in Europe (CANONIC STUDY) [3] and North America (NACSELD) [4]. As each continent (Europe, Asia, and North America) used its own definition, the World Congress of Gastroenterology subsequently suggested the following ACLF definition: "a syndrome in patients with chronic liver disease with or without previously diagnosed cirrhosis which is characterized by acute hepatic decompensation resulting in liver failure (jaundice and prolongation of the INR [International Normalized Ratio]) and one or more extrahepatic organ failures that is associated with increased mortality within a period of 28 days and up to 3 months from onset" [1]. Thus, the main difference between ACLF and decompensated cirrhosis is the development of organ failure. The difficulty in pediatrics is that organ failure cannot be based on absolute value (i.e., creatinine value or mean arterial pressure), as cut-off values are age-dependent. The SOFA (Sequential Organ Failure Assessment) Score has been used and validated for several years in adults patients admitted to ICU. This score has been modified to CLIF-SOFA, CLIF-C OF (Organ Failure) in patient with liver disease. A recent pediatric study, published in 2020, used a modified ACLF definition called p-CLIF in 11,300 children listed for liver transplant in the United States through the Organ Procurement and Transplantation Network [5]. In this study, renal failure was defined as a 60% elevation from the mean normal creatinine for that age group. The modified pediatric ACLF criteria are presented in Table 1.

> Acute-on-chronic liver failure is defined as an acute hepatic decompensation with liver failure and one or more extrahepatic organ failures.

Prevalence

In adult population, several multicenter studies have shown a prevalence of ACLF to be around 24–30% of hospitalized cirrhotic patients [3, 4, 6]. Of this, about 20% present with ACLF at admission and 10% will develop ACLF during hospitalization. Unfortunately, prevalence studies are limited in pediatrics, and given the lack of consensus regarding the definition of ACLF in Asia, Europe, and North America, as well as the absence of unified pediatric-specific criteria, prevalence of ACLF in children has been difficult to reconcile. Four studies describe ACLF prevalence in children with chronic liver disease, ranging from 12% to 47% [7–10]. Recently, when analyzing children on the waiting list for a liver transplantation at Chicago Hospital, it was found that 30% of patients develop ACLF, representing 12% of hospital admission for liver decompensation. Of those, 55% had biliary atresia [11]. Another pediatric multicenter study evaluating the database for Organ Procurement and Transplantation Network showed that 2.5% of the total listing corresponded to patients presenting with ACLF. Biliary atresia was again the most common etiology in ACLF group with 48% [5].

Etiology

Etiology of Chronic Liver Disease

ACLF is not limited to patients known to previously have compensated cirrhosis but may represent the first clinical manifestation of the liver disease. Two pediatric studies published in 2011 [12] and 2012 [13] showed that autoimmune hepatitis and Wilson disease were the most common underlying etiology for ACLF representing 22.2–41.9% and 27.7–41.9%, respectively. Now that this syndrome has been more defined, it seems that biliary atresia is probably the most common primary cause, representing nearly half of the cases [5, 11]. Pediatric liver pathologies with proclivity to have an ACLF are biliary atresia, other chronic cholestasis, including sclerosing cholangitis or PFIC (progressive familial intrahepatic cholestasis), autoimmune hepatitis, Wilson disease, other metabolic diseases, and obstructive venopathies. In cases of autoimmune hepatitis and Wilson disease, flare-up of the underlying disorder is a frequent cause of acute liver failure [14]. Less commonly, reactivation of hepatitis B, hepatitis C, or NASH, which have been well described in adult studies for ACLF, may also present in pediatric cases.

Etiology of the Acute Insult

The most frequent precipitating event in children with chronic liver disease is an infectious episode. The agents triggering organ failure are usually bacterial, causing infections such as cholangitis, spontaneous bacterial peritonitis, urinary tract infections, bacteremia or pneumonia, or viral leading to respiratory tract infections, pneumonia, or gastroenteritis. Viral causes such as parainfluenza, rhinovirus, CMV, influenza, and adenovirus have been identified as causes of ACLF in patients with biliary atresia [10]. In underdeveloped countries or Asia, reactivation of hepatitis B or superimposition of acute hepatitis A or hepatitis E on chronic liver disease are the predominant reasons of acute hepatic decompensation and organ failure. Fungal or parasitic infections are rarer but a possible precipitating factor. Among the noninfectious etiologies, alcoholic hepatitis, which is the most common factor in adult population in western countries [15], is rarely seen in pediatrics. However, acute hepatotoxicity can result from drugs or natural products through direct or idiosyncratic mechanisms of liver injury. Flare up of autoimmune hepatitis or Wilson Disease, possibly from noncompliance to medical treatment or a superimposed infectious or toxic injury, can result in acute liver failure. Less frequently, ACLF can occur as a consequence of a gastrointestinal bleeding or acute thrombosis.

Previous study, that did not include biliary atresia patients, showed that hepatotropic viral insult (37–94%), flare of autoimmune liver disease (9.6–17%), and flare of Wilson disease (0–27%) were the most common acute precipitating events [12, 13, 16]. In a recent cohort of children with biliary atresia, sepsis (45%) and gastrointestinal bleeding (40%) were the most common reasons for acute deterioration [10]. In about 5–10% of the cases, the acute insult is unidentifiable [17].

Pathogenesis

The pathophysiology of ACLF is not fully understood but there is growing evidence that ACLF has a distinct pathophysiological pathway compared to decompensated cirrhosis. This difference in pathophysiology may explain the increased mortality in ACLF compared to decompensated cirrhosis.

Patients with cirrhosis already exhibit baseline chronic systemic inflammation owing to intestinal dysbiosis, loss of integrity of the intestinal mucosal barrier, and intermittent translocations of pathogen-associated molecular patterns (PAMPs) [18–20]. Patients with ACLF present with an excessive systemic inflammatory response (SIRS), mainly shown by an increase of circulating neutrophils and of C-reactive protein (CRP) [21]. This "inflammatory storm" outbalances the baseline inflammation already present in patients with cirrhosis or acute decompensation without ACLF [22]. This immune overactivation may result in a relative weakness and ineffective reactions to microorganisms.

One of the hallmarks of ACLF is the high WBC count, which can be explained by the increase level of G-CSF being produced in the context of systemic inflammation. G-CSF is an important regulator and hematopoietic agent that promote differentiation and activation of neutrophils. Similarly to what has been observed in patients with sepsis, PAMPs released by the infecting bacteria lead to a remarkable increase of inflammatory markers (IL-6, IL-8, IL-17A, IL-22, IL-23R, TNFa, monocyte chemoattractant protein 1), vasodilatory molecules (Vascular Cell

Adhesion Molecule (VCAM), and Vascular Endothelial Growth Factor A (VEGFA)) and reactive oxygen species [23–26]. In patients with ACLF, the increase in pro-inflammatory cytokines and chemokines is higher than can be observed in patients with decompensated cirrhosis, being strongly associated with the severity of organ failure and 28- and 90-days mortality rates. Improvements are associated with lowering levels of IL-6 and IL-8 [23], whereas nonsurviving ACLF patients have higher IL-23R expression [27]. Concomitantly, anti-inflammatory cytokines, such as IL-10 and IL-1Ra, are secreted in patients with ACLF, but this seems to be insufficient to counteract the massive proinflammatory storm [23]. Other noninfectious precipitating events can cause SIRS, without sepsis, by the release of damage-associated molecular patterns (DAMPs) from the injured liver [28].

Mitochondrial dysfunction is also important in the development of organ failure and ACLF. Fibroblast Growth Factor 21 (FGF21), a peptide hormone secreted by the liver, is an important marker of mitochondrial dysfunction and is associated with anti-inflammatory properties. In patients that show sign of ACLF or in those that subsequently develop this syndrome after admission, FGF21 levels were found to be high but did not correlate with the severity of the disorder [29]. Level of FGF21 is independent of the cause of liver disease, precipitating event, or genetic background. In other terms, FGF21 could be a predictive marker of ACLF development and a tool to initiate earlier and rigorous treatment or follow-up for these patients.

In conclusion, organ failure in ACLF result from the direct deleterious effects of the overactivated innate immune system on the microcirculation and tissue cell homeostasis as well as mitochondrial dysfunction.

Natural History and Outcome of ACLF

Liver failure is central in the clinical picture, and the most frequent complications are ascites, hepatic encephalopathy, increase bilirubin level, and renal failure. These patients show a hypocoagulable status, correlating with systemic inflammation and survival rate but not with bleeding rates [30].

Limited data are available on the natural history of ACLF, but according to the CLIF consortium of 388 adult patients, resolution or improvement of ACLF was seen in approximately half of the patients, whereas 30% had a steady or fluctuating course and 20% worsened [1]. It is, however, well accepted that ACLF carries a worse prognosis than acute decompensation, and thus, patients admitted with ACLF are less likely to be discharged home (22% vs. 91%) and more likely to die or receive a liver transplant [11]. Additionally, mortality is associated with the number of organ failure. A study done in the USA on 66 children showed a mortality rate of 0% with 1 organ failure, 29% with 2 organ failures, 33% with 3 organ failures, and 66% with 4 organ failures [11]. As compared to adults, this study also showed that respiratory failure was more common in children, developing in 74% of them, and renal failure was the least common with 30% incidence. Respiratory failure may result from pulmonary infections, pulmonary edema, pleura effusion, or acute respiratory distress syndrome but mechanical ventilation might be required for airway protections in cases of variceal bleeding or hepatic encephalopathy. In adult studies, more than half developed renal failure whereas respiratory failure was seen in less than 2% of ACLF patients [3]. Another pediatric study revealed that one in five patients with autoimmune hepatitis and Wilson disease, presenting as ACLF, developed renal failure; such complication being associated with a worst prognosis in those patients [31].

Acute kidney injury (AKI), which usually develops 4 weeks after onset of ACLF, is a consequence of hepatorenal syndrome (HRS) or sepsis in one-third of cases, of nephrotoxic drugs in nearly one-fourth of cases, of dehydration in 10% of cases, and occasionally results from acute tubular necrosis secondary to bile pigment [31]. Higher baseline bilirubin >300 μmol/L and the presence of systemic inflammatory response syndrome (SIRS) were risk factors for the development of AKI. Outcome was considerably worse in patients with AKI compared to those who did not develop AKI, with a probability of dying or requiring liver transplant 7.7 times higher. This probability was higher when AKI was secondary to HRS and lower when related to drug-induced kidney failure, but etiology of liver disease did not affect outcome [31].

Several adult studies have shown that higher MELD score, lower baseline mean arterial pressure, higher bilirubin, need for mechanical ventilation, and even lower baseline hemoglobin were associated with higher risk of developing ACLF in the following year [32, 33]. In one pediatric study, clinical factors associated with ACLF development were increased creatinine, AST, INR, and positive blood culture, when compared with patients on the waiting list who were hospitalized without organ failures [11]. Another study on biliary atresia showed that increased bilirubin levels at 3 months and increased INR at 6 months post-portoenterostomy were associated with the development of ACLF [10]. As patients with ACLF develop organ failures, they are more likely to be admitted to PICU and length of stay in ICU was 20 times longer in patients with ACLF compared to those who did not develop organ failure (13 days vs. 0.6 days). Overall hospitalization was also 3 times longer (24.3 days vs. 7.9 days) [11].

As mentioned previously, ACLF is characterized by high mortality rate which depends on the number of failing organs. In adult series, 90-days mortality is between 30–50% of patients, reaching more than 70% in cases with three organ failures [3, 4]. This is in contrast to acute decompensation without organ failure that only has a 2–3% mortality. White blood cells count and response to treatment are additional predictor factors to the grade of ACLF, for 90-day mortality [34].

Predictive Models and Mortality

Model for end-stage liver disease (MELD) is usually used for prognostication and for guiding therapy in patient with liver disease. However, this score does not take into account cerebral, circulatory and respiratory failure and show poor sensitivity for predicting outcomes in ACLF patients. Organ dysfunction models used in intensive care units, such as SOFA (Sequential Organ Failure Assessment), have previously been used in assessing critically sick adult cirrhotics, as it evaluates six different organ functions (respiratory, cardiovascular, hepatic, renal, neurological, and coagulation). Unfortunately, SOFA showed poor diagnostic accuracy in patients with ACLF, thus prognosticating scores were modified for CLIF-SOFA (Chronic Liver Failure - Sequential Organ Failure Assessment) and CLIF-C OFs (CLIF Consortium Organ Failure score) [35, 36], in order to discriminate patients likely to die, to offer timely liver transplant or to prevent unnecessary liver transplant in those likely to survive with their native liver. CLIF-C ACLFs (CLIF Consortium ACLF score) is a mathematical model that includes CLIF-C OFs as well as age and white blood cell count. This scoring system was found to be a better predictor of outcomes in patients with ACLF compared to MELD, MELD-Na, or APACHE II score [35]. As patients may improve, worsen, or fluctuate in the first few days, scoring done at day 3–7 after the development of ACLF, predicted the 28- and 90-day mortality significantly better than scoring done at diagnosis [37]. Eighty percent of patients achieved their final ACLF grade 3–7 days after onset. This score, done at day 3–7, could be used for continuing supportive management, listing urgently or to withdraw care owing to futility. AARC (Asian Pacific-ACLF Research Consortium) is an alternative score that can easily be done at bedside and the Asian Pacific association for the study of the liver (APASL) [17] suggested an algorithm for management based on the evolution of the score and grade of ACLF. Score 5–7 corresponds to ACLF grade 1, score 8–10 to grade 2, and score 11–15 to grade 3. Score <10 at presentation or a decrease in score below 10 by the end of first week is associated with higher chance of survival. Patients with AARC Score >10 or those who did not show improvement with a 2-points decrease after 7 days, should be listed for liver transplant. If the score is >11 with more than two extra-hepatic organ failures and no improvement after 1 week, supportive or withdrawal of care might be considered at it is associated with very poor prognosis, and liver transplant would possibly be futile [17]. Again, the AARC score was found to be superior to MELD, MELD-Na, and CLIF-SOFA [38].

In children, mortality has been estimated around 30%, and scores such as AARC-ACLF (Asian Pacific-ACLF Research Consortium) and CLIF-SOFA are used for prognosis (see Tables 2 and 3). Both prognostic scores were more accurate to predict outcome than PELD, CTP, PRISM III, PELOD 2, and APACHE III [39].

Table 2 Asian Pacific acute-on-chronic liver failure Research Consortium (AARC-ACLF) pediatric severity score

Scoring system	1	2	3
Total bilirubin (μmol/L)	<256	256–427	>427
Creatinine (rise from baseline)	<1.5×	1.5–3×	>3× or need for RRT
HE grade	0	1–2	3–4
INR	<1.8	1.8–2.5	>2.5
Lactate (mmol/L)	<1.5	1.5–2.5	>2.5

HE Hepatic encephalopathy, *RRT* Renal replacement therapy

Table 3 CLIF-SOFA pediatric severity score

Organ system	0	1	2	3	4
Liver (bilirubin, µmol/L)	<20	21–34	35–102	103–205	>206
Kidney (rise in baseline creatinine)	<1.5×	1.5–2×	2–3×	>3×	Need for RRT
Cerebral (HE grade)	0	1	2	3	4
Coagulation (INR)	<1.1	1.1–1.25	1.26–1.5	1.51–2.5	>2.5
Circulation (systolic BP)	Normal for age	<5th centile for age	Norepi <0.5 µg/kg/min	Norepi >0.5 µg/kg/min	Norepi >0.5 µg/kg/min and second inotrope
Respiratory (PaO_2/FiO_2)	>400	301–400	201–300	101–200	<100

BP Blood pressure, *HE* Hepatic encephalopathy, *RRT* Renal replacement therapy

Pediatric modification of AARC-ACLF and CLIF-SOFA scores were as effective as their original scores and both scores were equivalent; however, AARC-ACLF is probably easier to use. Children with AARC-ACLF and CLIF-SOFA score of less than 11 indicated a relatively good outcome, but if above 11, they become candidate for urgent liver transplant, as it predicted poor outcome in 85% [39]. As evolution is dynamic, a rising score is also an indicator of high mortality. AARC-ACLF score of 5–7, 8–10 and >11 were associated with 28-day mortality of 12.7%, 44.5%, and 85.9%, respectively [39].

In a group of children, mainly with diagnosis of autoimmune hepatitis and Wilson disease, poor outcome at 90 days was observed in around 40% of patients, 30.4% died, and 8.9% received a liver transplant. In this cohort, encephalopathy grades 3 or 4 was associated with a poor outcome, as well as high bilirubin, INR >3.5, or two or more organ failures [16]. This would likely be reflected as AARC-ACLF or CLIFF-SOFA score more than 11.

In the post-liver transplant course, patients with ACLF also tend to have prolonged ICU course and slightly worse outcome than patients who received liver transplant in a compensated stable status. A study on 99 children with biliary atresia showed that PICU length of stay was 7 days vs. 2 days in ACLF vs. non-ACLF [10].

Management

There are no specific treatments for ACLF but management is rather supportive. Treatment should be directed at the precipitating event, preventing secondary injury or complications, lessening the inflammatory response, and supporting failing organs. The majority of patients will require intensive care management for organ support (mechanical ventilation, renal replacement therapy, vasopressors) and thus, prompt recognition and transfer to ICU with a liver transplant center will reduce mortality [21].

Initial steps are aimed at addressing the acute insult and thus thorough investigations must be carried out on admission. Use of early broad-spectrum antibiotics for suspected or proven infections, upper GI bleeding, or worsening hepatic encephalopathy is vital. Choice of empirical antibiotic should be based on local resistance profiles, environment, severity, and type of infection. Patients with spontaneous bacterial peritonitis may receive blood volume expansion with albumin on top of antibiotics. Administration of antiviral therapy for reactivation of hepatitis B [40], new infection with hepatitis E, and keeping a low threshold for antifungal therapy lead to improved survival. As bacterial infections can both be a trigger of ACLF and a complication of ACLF, protocols for prophylaxis should be considered in each case [24]. Up to 46% of patients with ACLF not triggered by infections, presented with bacterial infection during follow-up. The risk of secondary complication with bacterial infections was directly associated with the grade of ACLF [24]. Therapeutic endoscopy and blood transfusion may be required when the acute decompensation is secondary to upper GI bleeding.

Management is also directed toward supporting the declining organs. Treatment of AKI in ACLF depends on the etiology, severity, and complications and includes bilirubin reduction, avoidance of nephrotoxic drugs, volume expansion with fluids or albumin, and maintaining good mean arterial pressure [31]. In patients with hepato-renal syndrome, treatment with terlipressin and albumin (1 g/kg/day) can be used [34]. In case of renal failure, electrolytes imbalance (such as hyperkalemia or hyponatremia) or oliguria resulting in severe volume overload, renal replacement therapy may be needed, if the patient is not responding to conservative management. Hepatic encephalopathy is treated with ammonia-lowering agents such as lactulose, rifaximin, and nitrogen scavengers or renal replacement therapy in severe cases. Circulatory failure is managed with fluid administration, vasopressors support such as noradrenaline, dopamine, or terlipressin and hydrocortisone in refractory states, whereas mechanical ventilation is used for respiratory failure [32].

Prompt recognition of underlying liver disease in patients unknown to have chronic liver disease previously is also important. Recognizing flare-up of autoimmune hepatitis or Wilson disease to establish early immunosuppressive or chelating treatment is mandatory. Plamapheresis may be considered in those patients if first-line treatment is ineffective.

Extracorporeal liver support systems such as MARS (molecular adsorbent recirculating system) [41], ELAD (extracorporeal liver assist device]) [42], or fractionated plasma separation and adsorption system [43] did not show survival benefit in ACLF patients compared to standard therapy, despite transient improvement in hepatorenal syndrome, encephalopathy, circulatory dysfunction, or immune dysfunction.

ACLF is a high mortality condition, it is therefore important to provide timely supportive management but also to consider salvage liver transplantation (LT), as an option. As waitlist mortality is high and steady for patients with ACLF and exceeds that of patients with acute liver failure (ALF) at 61 days (Fig. 1a) [5], early listing for liver transplant should be done, after recognition of ACLF, as irreversible organ failure can compromise transplantation. In an ideal situation, liver transplantation

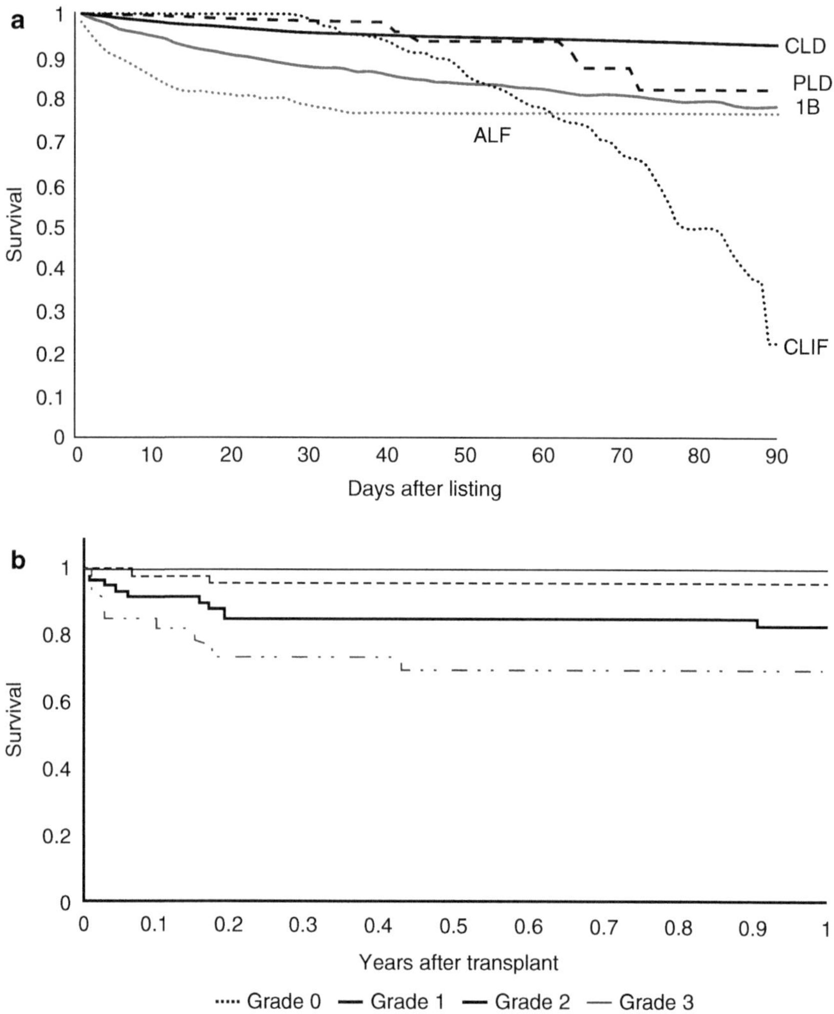

Fig. 1 Waitlist Kaplan-Meier survival to 90 days (Panel **a**). Posttransplant survival versus ACLF grade at transplant in p-CLIF patients (Panel **b**). (**a**) Demonstrates the difference in mortality between liver failure groups. The ALF group demonstrates high early mortality that plateaus by 38 days. Both ACLF groups have a steep, steady mortality rate that surpasses the mortality curve for ALF at 61 days. Only 22.2% of patients meeting our p-CLIF criteria survive to 90 days without transplant. Survival at 90 days is above 75% for CLD, PLD. (**b**) Depicts posttransplant survival compared with CLIF grade at transplant. ACLF - acute-on-chronic liver failure, CLIF - chronic liver failure, p-CLIF - pediatric CLIF, CLD - Chronic liver disease, PLD - progressive liver disease. (Source with permission: Godfrey et al. [5])

should be offered to patients with low prognostic scores and as soon as possible, since progression of organ failures such as that of respiratory and brain were highly predictive of delisting or death [44]. In a patient with ACLF grade 2, the window period for liver transplant might only be 1–2 weeks long before the patient becomes too sick for LT. Contraindications to liver transplant in patients with ACLF are:

presence of cerebral edema, intracranial bleeding, active uncontrolled infection, hemodynamic instability, and possibly the need for mechanical ventilation [2]. In adult patients, it was recently shown that even with high ACLF grade, LT is feasible and showed excellent results [45]. Nevertheless, it should be mentioned that even in patients who survive after LT, they require longer period in the ICU post-transplant. Adult data from the CANONIC study showed that the 1-year probability of survival post-transplant in ACLF patients was slightly lower than that of the overall population receiving an LT (75% vs. 88% respectively) [37]. A recent pediatric study, looking at the USA Organ Procurement and Transplantation Network database [5], including 11,300 children listed for liver failure, showed more promising data. The mortality rate is slightly greater in the 90 days post-transplant in ACLF patients compared to all other types of liver failure, but the 90–365 days survival rate is comparable. The post-transplant death in ACLF seems to be clustered in the first 90 days and having two or more organ failures pre-transplant is associated with decreased survival (Fig. 1b). Biliary atresia being the leading etiology of chronic liver disease in children accounts for 45% of ACLF list, but is protective against mortality post-transplant.

It must be recognized that many issues concerning LT remain unresolved in this group of patients notably: (1) pre-LT assessment, (2) defining good timing for listing and transplanting, (3) how to efficiently support patients in the waiting list, and (4) causes of delisting [21].

Liver transplant is probably the only cure in ACLF patients. There are very few alternatives, at present, to LT but granulocytes colony-stimulating factor (G-CSF) can help in hepatic regeneration by activating bone marrow-derived CD34+ cells, reducing the occurrence of sepsis and subsequent multiorgan failure development. Its use, combined with darbopoietin alpha, was associated with improved survival rate at 1 year compared to placebo, (68.6% vs. 26.7%), and reduced risk of septic shock at follow-up (6.9% vs. 38.5%) [46].

In a patient with ACLF grade 2, the window period for liver transplant might only be 1–2 weeks long before the patient becomes too sick for liver transplantation.

Conclusions

ACLF is an increasingly recognized entity, being associated with a high mortality rate, 10–15 times higher than patients with chronic liver disease and acute decompensation. Pathogenesis is associated with uncontrolled inflammatory response leading to multi-organ failure. Recognition of the trigger causes of this syndrome would allow establishing protocols for its prevention; representing a great economy in health care costs and in human lives. Susceptibility to developing an acute complication is related to the liver function failure, circulatory dysfunction and low hemoglobin levels. The presence of kidney failure and its degree as well as other organ failures influence the outcome negatively. Pediatric AARC-ACLF and CLIF-SOFA scores >11 are associated with poor prognosis and thus liver transplantation should be decided rapidly and carried out in the first weeks after the onset, to reduce mortality. Organ allocations score or consensus for deceased donor allocations priority need to be modified to favor urgent transplant in patients with ACLF as waitlist mortality is much higher in those patients compared to CLD or ALF after 61 days. Liver transplant is potentially the only curative treatment option, irrespective of etiology, with 1-year survival rate similar to other LT recipients (CLD, acute decompensation, or ALF).

References

1. Jalan R, Yurdaydin C, Bajaj JS, et al. Toward an improved definition of acute-on-chronic liver failure. Gastroenterology. 2014;147:4–10.
2. Sarin SK, Kumar A, Almeida JA, et al. Acute-on-chronic liver failure: consensus recommendations of the Asian Pacific Association for the study of the liver (APASL). Hepatol Int. 2009;3:269–82.
3. Moreau R, Jalan R, Gines P, et al.; for CANONIC Study Investigators of the EASL–CLIF Consortium. Acute-on-chronic liver failure is a distinct syndrome that develops in patients with acute decompensation of cirrhosis. Gastroenterology. 2013;144:1426–37.
4. Bajaj JS, O'Leary JG, Reddy KR, et al.; for North American Consortium for the Study of End-Stage Liver Disease (NACSELD). Survival in infection related acute-on-chronic liver failure is defined by extrahepatic organ failures. Hepatology. 2014;60:250–6.
5. Godfrey E, Desai M, Lam F, et al. Higher waitlist mortality in pediatric acute on chronic liver failure in the UNOS database. J Pediatr Gastroenterol Nutr. 2021;72:80–7.
6. Sargenti K, Prytz H, Nilsson E, et al. Predictors of mortality among patients with compensated and decompensated liver cirrhosis: the role of bacterial infections and infection-related acute-on- chronic liver failure. Scand J Gastroenterol. 2015;50(7):875–83.
7. Bolia R, Srivastava A, Marak R, et al. Role of procalcitonin and creactive protein as biomarkers of infection in children with liver disease. J Pediatr Gastroenterol Nutr. 2016;63:406–11.
8. Bolia R, Srivastava A, Marak R, et al. Prevalence and impact of bacterial infections in children with liver disease-a prospective study. J Clin Exp Hepatol. 2018;8:35–41.
9. Bolia R, Srivastava A, Yachha SK, et al. Pediatric CLIF-SOFA score is the best predictor of 28-day mortality in children with decompensated chronic liver disease. J Hepatol. 2018;68:449–55.
10. D'Souza R, Grammatikopoulos T, Pradhan A, et al. Acute-on-chronic liver failure in children with biliary atresia awaiting liver transplantation. Pediatr Transplant. 2019;23:e13339.
11. Banc-Husu AM, Neighbors K, Rychlik K, et al. Admission characteristics identify risk of pediatric acute-on-chronic liver failure. J Pediatr Gastroenterol Nutr. 2020;70:783–8.
12. Lal J, Thapa BR, Rawal P, et al. Predictors of outcome in acute-on-chronic liver failure in children. Hepatol Int. 2011;5(2):693–7.
13. Jagadisan B, Srivastava A, Yachha SK, Poddar U. Acute on chronic liver disease in children from the developing world: recognition and prognosis. J Pediatr Gastroenterol Nutr. 2012;54(1):77–82.
14. Di Giorgio A, Nicastro E, Dalla Rosa D, Nebbia G, Sonzogni A, D'Antiga L. Transplant-free survival in chronic liver disease presenting as acute liver failure in childhood. Transplantation. 2019;103(3):544–51.

15. Moreau R, Arroyo V. Acute-on-chronic liver failure: a new clinical entity. Clin Gastroenterol Hepatol. 2015;13(5):836–41.
16. Alam S, Lal BB, Sood V, Rawat D. Pediatric acute-on-chronic liver failure in a specialized liver unit: prevalence, profile, outcome and predictive factors. J Pediatr Gastroenterol Nutr. 2016;63(4):400–5.
17. Sarin SK, Choudhury A, Sharma MK, Maiwall R, Al Mahtab M, et al. Acute-on-chronic liver failure: consensus recommendations of the Asian Pacific association for the study of the liver (APASL): an update. Hepatol Int. 2019;13(4):353–90.
18. Bernardi M, Moreau R, Angeli P, et al. Mechanisms of decompensation and organ failure in cirrhosis: from peripheral arterial vasodilation to systemic inflammation hypothesis. J Hepatol. 2015;63:1272–84.
19. Wiest R, Lawson M, Geuking M. Pathological bacterial translocation in liver cirrhosis. J Hepatol. 2014;60:197–209.
20. Albillos A, Lario M, Álvarez-Mon M. Cirrhosis-associated immune dysfunction:distinctive features and clinical relevance. J Hepatol. 2014;61:1385–96.
21. Putignano A, Gustot T. New concepts in acute-on-chronic liver failure: implications for liver transplantation. Liver Transpl. 2017;23(2):234–43.
22. Jalan R, Gines P, Olson JC, Mookerjee RP, Moreau R, Garcia-Tsao G, Arroyo V, Kamath PS. Acute-on chronic liver failure. J Hepatol. 2012;57(6):1336–48.
23. Clària J, Arroyo V, Moreau R. The acute-on-chronic liver failure syndrome, or when the innate immune system goes astray. J Immunol. 2016;197(10):3755–61.
24. Fernández J, Acevedo J, Wiest R, Gustot T, Amoros A, et al. Bacterial and fungal infections in acute-on-chronic liver failure: prevalence, characteristics and impact on prognosis. Gut. 2018;67(10):1870–80.
25. Clària J, Stauber RE, Coenraad MJ, et al. Systemic inflammation in decompensated cirrhosis: characterization and role in acute-on-chronic liver failure. Hepatology. 2016;64:1249–64.
26. Gandoura S, Weiss E, Rautou PE, et al. Gene- and exon-expression profiling reveals an extensive LPS-induced response in immune cells in patients with cirrhosis. J Hepatol. 2013;58:936–48.
27. Khanam A, Trehanpati N, Sarin SK. Increased interleukin-23 receptor (IL-23R) expression is associated with disease severity in acute-on-chronic liver failure. Liver Int. 2019;39(6):1062–70.
28. Kubes P, Mehal WZ. Sterile inflammation in the liver. Gastroenterology. 2012;143:1158–72.
29. Ruiz-Margáin A, Pohlmann A, Ryan P, Schierwagen R, Chi-Cervera LA, et al. Fibroblast growth factor 21 is an early predictor of acute-on-chronic liver failure in critically ill patients with cirrhosis. Liver Transpl. 2018;24(5):595–605.
30. Blasi A, Calvo A, Prado V, Reverter E, Reverter JC, et al. Coagulation failure in patients with acute-on-chronic liver failure and decompensated cirrhosis: beyond the international normalized ratio. Hepatology. 2018;68(6):2325–37.
31. Lal BB, Alam S, Sood V, Rawat D, Khanna R. Profile, risk factors and outcome of acute kidney injury in paediatric acute-on-chronic liver failure. Liver Int. 2018;38(10):1777–84.
32. Piano S, Tonon M, Vettore E, Stanco M, Pilutti C, et al. Incidence, predictors and outcomes of acute-on-chronic liver failure in outpatients with cirrhosis. J Hepatol. 2017;67(6):1177–84.
33. Levesque E, Saliba F, Ichaï P, Samuel D. Outcome of patients with cirrhosis requiring mechanical ventilation in ICU. J Hepatol. 2014;60(3):570–8.
34. Piano S, Schmidt HH, Ariza X, Amoros A, Romano A, et al. EASL CLIF Consortium, European Foundation for the Study of Chronic Liver Failure (EF Clif). Association between grade of acute on chronic liver failure and response to terlipressin and albumin in patients with hepatorenal syndrome. Clin Gastroenterol Hepatol. 2018;16(11):1792–1800.e3.
35. Jalan R, Saliba F, Pavesi M, Amoros A, Moreau R, Gine's P, et al. Development and validation of a prognostic score to predict mortality in patients with acute-on-chronic liver failure. J Hepatol. 2014;61:1038–47.
36. Zheng YX, Zhong X, Li YJ, Fan XG. Performance of scoring systems to predict mortality of patients with acute-on-chronic liver failure: a systematic review and meta-analysis. J Gastroenterol Hepatol. 2017;32(10):1668–78.

37. Gustot T, Fernandez J, Garcia E, Morando F, Caraceni P, et al. CANONIC study investigators of the EASL-CLIF consortium. Clinical course of acute-on-chronic liver failure syndrome and effects on prognosis. Hepatology. 2015;62(1):243–52.
38. Choudhury A, Jindal A, for the APASL ACLF Working Party, et al. Liver failure determines the outcome in patients of acute-on-chronic liver failure (ACLF)-comparison of APASL-ACLF research consortium (AARC) and CLIF-SOFA model. Hepatol Int. 2017;11(5):461–71.
39. Lal BB, Sood V, Khanna R, Alam S. How to identify the need for liver transplantation in pediatric acute-on-chronic liver failure? Hepatol Int. 2018;12(6):552–9.
40. Garg H, Sarin SK, Kumar M, Garg V, Sharma BC, Kumar A. Tenofovir improves the outcome in patients with spontaneous reactivation of hepatitis B presenting as acute-on-chronic liver failure. Hepatology. 2011;53(3):774–80.
41. Banares R, Nevens F, Larsen FS, Jalan R, Albillos A, et al.; for RELIEF Study Group. Extracorporeal albumin dialysis with the molecular adsorbent recirculating system in acute-on-chronic liver failure: the RELIEF trial. Hepatology. 2013;57:1153–62.
42. Thompson JA, Subramanian R, Al-Khafaji A, Reich DJ, Nicholas RM, et al. The effect of extracorporeal C3a cellular therapy in severe alcoholic hepatitis – the ELAD trial. Hepatology. 2015;62(Suppl 6):1379A.
43. Kribben A, Gerken G, Haag S, Herget-Rosenthal S, Treichel U, et al.; for HELIOS Study Group. Effects of fractionated plasma separation and adsorption on survival in patients with acute-on-chronic liver failure. Gastroenterology. 2012;142:782–9.
44. Reddy KR, O'Leary JG, Kamath PS, Fallon MB, Biggins SW, et al.; for North American Consortium for the Study of End-Stage Liver Disease. High risk of delisting or death in liver transplant candidates following infections: results from the North American consortium for the study of end-stage liver disease. Liver Transpl. 2015;21:881–8.
45. Arroyo V. Acute-on-chronic liver failure in cirrhosis requires expedited decisions for liver transplantation. Gastroenterology. 2019;156(5):1248–9.
46. Kedarisetty CK, Anand L, Bhardwaj A, et al. Combination of granulocyte colony-stimulating factor and erythropoietin improves outcomes of patients with decompensated cirrhosis. Gastroenterology. 2015;148:1362–70.e7.

Liver Failure and the Brain

Genevieve Du Pont Thibodeau and Laurence Ducharme Crevier

Hepatic encephalopathy (HE) refers to an alteration of normal brain function in the context of acute or chronic liver failure. HE includes a wide range of neurological symptoms of which intracranial hypertension and coma are the most concerning complications.

Pathophysiology

Hyperammonia

Hyperammonia in the central nervous system (CNS) arises either from diffusion from the blood and cerebrospinal fluid or from in situ production from the metabolism of endogenous nitrogen-containing substances. The role of ammonia in the pathophysiology of HE is not fully understood but has been the focus of multiple studies. In acute liver failure, there is an imperfect correlation between plasmatic ammonia level and the severity of HE, nonetheless higher levels of ammonia (>200 μmol/L) are associated with worse neurological dysfunction and morbidity [1]. In the CNS, removal of ammonia is exclusively dependent on the activity of glutamine synthetase, a cytosolic enzyme that converts ammonia and glutamate into glutamine ($Glutamate + ATP + NH_3 \rightarrow Glutamine + ADP + Phosphate$). Glutamine synthetase is primarily located in astrocytes [2]. It already functions at near-maximal capacity under normal physiologic conditions. Its activity can be easily saturated

G. D. P. Thibodeau (✉) · L. D. Crevier
Pediatric Intensive Care Unit, Department of Pediatrics, CHU Sainte-Justine, Université de Montréal, Montreal, QC, Canada
e-mail: genevieve.du.pont-thibodeau.med@ssss.gouv.qc.ca; laurence.ducharme.crevier.med@ssss.gouv.qc.ca

P. Jouvet, F. Alvarez (eds.), *Liver Diseases in the Pediatric Intensive Care Unit*,
https://doi.org/10.1007/978-3-030-79132-2_4

and hyperammonemia can consequently rapidly develop. Ammonia influences the passage of different molecules across the blood brain barrier (BBB), including the passage of amino acids, affecting brain catecholamine synthesis and inducing production of false neurotransmitters resulting in impaired GABAergic, serotonergic, and glutamatergic neurotransmission [3].

Glutamine

Glutamine is a neutral amino acid that contributes to ammonia detoxification in the CNS (end-product of ammonia detoxification). Glutamine synthesis by astrocytes partially protects neurons during increases of blood ammonia concentrations, resulting in increased intracellular levels of glutamine. This high level of glutamine in the CNS ultimately results in astrocyte swelling and cytotoxic cerebral edema [4]. Once glutamine is produced in the astrocyte, it is liberated via the sodium-coupled neutral amino acid transporter (SNAT5) into the extracellular space. Animal studies suggest that one mechanism driving the cerebral edema in acute liver failure is the downregulation of SNAT5 in astrocyte, thereby limiting the transfer of glutamine out of the astrocyte [5]. Furthermore, glutamine in the mitochondria induces the production of intracellular ammonia via the phosphate-activated glutaminase (PAG), which leads to mitochondrial dysfunction, free radicals production, and ultimately energy failure [4, 6].

Blood Brain Barrier (BBB)

HE is characterized by cerebral hyperemia, which is thought to be secondary to vasodilation and alteration of the BBB [7, 8]. Increased BBB permeability plays a major role in the physiopathology of HE [9, 10]. Blood brain barrier permeability may increase due to altered intercellular tight junctions and inflammation, leading to vasogenic edema and increased influx of ammonia to the brain [9]. Astrocyte swelling and dysfunction caused by glutamine entrapment further contributes to the alteration in tight junctions and BBB permeability. Inflammation appears to be a key element of HE. The breakdown of injured and necrotic hepatocytes releases numerous cytokines that contribute to systemic inflammation and vasodilation (TNF-α, IL-1, IL-6, interferon, ammonia) [11].

Ammonia exists in the gaseous (NH_3) and ionic (NH4+) forms. The ionic form does not cross the BBB due to its electric charge, whereas the gaseous form diffuses freely through the BBB. Hyperammonemia in ALF leads to higher passage of ammonia through BBB. At physiological pH levels, the proportion of the gaseous form (NH_3) is rather small [12]. Alkalosis favors a larger proportion of the gaseous and diffusible NH_3 form, whereas acidosis favors higher level of ionic, nondiffusible ammonia. It is interesting to note that many patients with HE hyperventilate, which favors the diffusion of NH_3 through the BBB. The physiological versus pathological nature of this phenomenon remains unclear.

Glutamate

The increased production of glutamine leads to excess of extracellular glutamate (via the glutamate-glutamine cycle) [5]. Glutamate is the main excitatory neurotransmitter, and alteration in the glutamatergic pathways is likely to affect numerous CNS functions. Release of glutamate from the pre-synaptic neuron into the extracellular space activates the ionotropic glutamate receptors in the synaptic membrane [13]. This excessive activation of N-Methyl-D-aspartic acid (NMDA) receptors leads to pathological excitotoxicity, which is characterized by the release of intracellular calcium, nitric oxide (NO) production, neuronal degeneration, and ultimately cellular death. In ALF, there is an imbalance between excitatory and inhibitory neurotransmission.

Cerebral Autoregulation

Autoregulation refers to the ability of the cerebral vascular system to maintain a constant cerebral blood flow by vasodilating and vasoconstricting in response to variations in systemic blood pressure. Impaired autoregulation has been described in patients with HE. Cerebral vasodilatation as is described in patients with HE also increases cerebral blood flow and causes further cerebral edema [14]. Elevation of extracellular glutamate levels activates NMDA receptors and through a cascade of events activates the neuronal nitric oxide synthase (nNOS), resulting in an increased production of nitric oxide (NO) contributing to vasodilation [15].

Cerebral Edema

Cerebral edema is thought to occur when large amounts of ammonia cross the blood brain barrier and combine with glutamate to form glutamine within the astrocytes. Glutamine is thought to induce a strong osmotic shift of fluid causing the astrocytes to swell. Furthermore, impaired autoregulation and cerebral vasodilatation can also increase cerebral blood flow and cause further intracranial hypertension [16, 17].

> Molecules diffusing through the BBB, and others produced in the brain, in association with brain loss of vascular regulation, contribute to central nervous system symptoms and signs observed in patients with acute liver failure.

Epidemiology and Clinical Presentation of HE

Hepatic encephalopathy is the most common complication affecting up to 38.6% of children with ALF and is an important predictor of outcome [18]. Hepatic encephalopathy is characterized by a spectrum of behavioral, cognitive, neurological, and electroencephalographic (EEG) abnormalities. It is categorized into five clinical stages called the West Haven criteria, which have prognostic values and range from minimal or no evidence of neurological dysfunction (stage 0) to overt coma (stage 4) (Table 1) [19, 20]. This classification was created to grade patients' mental state and to evaluate severity and progression of disease. The development of HE in infants and young children can be subtle on presentation and difficult to differentiate from other causes of altered mental status. In older children and adults, cognitive findings can include attention deficits, delayed reaction time, and impaired working memory. Sleep disturbance (insomnia or hypersomnia) is a common initial presentation and is often followed by mood changes, disorientation, inappropriate behavior, and confusion. Patients may develop neuromuscular impairment: bradykinesia, asterixis, ataxia, hyperreflexia, nystagmus, and/or slurred speech [21]. Some patients go on to develop overt intracranial hypertension and some may experience generalized, focal, or nonconvulsive seizures. Focal neurologic deficits have been reported in adults of which the most common is hemiplegia [22]. Patients with grade I-II HE rarely develop cerebral edema as opposed to those with higher grade HE. Cerebral edema tends to occur in the last stages of hepatic encephalopathy (stage III or IV) and can deteriorate rapidly to herniation and brain death. Cerebral edema occurs in 25–35% in patients with grade III HE and 65% to 75% in patients with grade IV HE. Only 25% of children with HE grade III or IV will spontaneously recover [18, 23].

Table 1 West Haven criteria

Grade 1	Mild lack of awareness
	Shortened attention span
Grade II	Lethargy
	Disorientation
	Inappropriate behavior
	Slurred speech
	Obvious asterixis
Grade III	Somnolent but arousable
	Gross disorientation
	Bizarre behavior
	Muscular rigidity
	Clonus
	Hyperreflexia
Grade IV	Coma
	Decerebrate posturing

Diagnosis, Monitoring, and Prognosis

Cerebral edema in patients with ALF is life-threatening. Some technical modalities may help in diagnosis and management. The current West Haven criteria help in grading severity of HE based on a series of clinical signs. Some neuromarkers (serum S100β and IL-6) are associated with the occurrence of HE in pediatric liver failure and therefore may contribute to the neurological assessment in ALF [24]. Ultrasound-guided measurement of optic nerve sheath diameter is a new technique that has the potential to help with HE assessment. It may correlate with HE progression and may therefore be useful for HE diagnosis and therapy adjustment [25]. Bispectral index electroencephalography (BIS) helps further discriminate HE grade I to IV [26]. Head computed tomography (CT) can help in detecting signs of intracranial hypertension by presenting radiologic findings of cerebral edema, compression of basal cisterns, mass effect, midline shift, and hydrocephalus. However, the absence of these radiological signs does not eliminate the presence of intracranial hypertension. Computed tomography is thus mainly used to exclude other causes of ongoing intracranial processes such as a mass or bleeding and is not routinely performed solely to diagnose intracranial hypertension [27]. Transcranial Doppler (TCD) is a noninvasive monitoring tool that measures the blood flow velocities of the major intracranial vessels. It can be useful in patients with HE to evaluate cerebral blood flow and assess cerebral autoregulation integrity. In patients with ALF cerebral edema, autoregulation is often impaired which can lead to increases in cerebral blood flow and subsequent cerebral edema. Increases in cerebral blood flow velocities as measured with TCDs have been shown to predict increased intracranial pressure. High cerebral blood flow has been associated with a poorer prognosis [28–30]. Disease progression with respect to cerebral perfusion has been described [30]. In mild stages of ALF, normal velocities are observed. As the disease progresses, increasing cerebral blood flow velocities underline an increase in cerebral blood flow and cerebral vasodilation, and when hemodynamic worsen, a sharply defined systolic flow peak at lower peak velocity is seen (Fig. 1). Finally, in the final stage of disease progression, a very sharp systolic peak with probable retrograde flow during diastole highlights severe intracranial pressure and poor cerebral perfusion.

> Transcranial Doppler is a noninvasive monitoring tool that measures the blood flow velocities of the major intracranial vessels. It can be useful in patients with severe HE to evaluate cerebral blood flow and assess cerebral autoregulation integrity.

Invasive intracranial pressure (ICP) monitoring is the most reliable tool to diagnose increased intracranial pressure. It can help with diagnosis, monitoring, as well as help guide and titrate specific management. Therapies targeting ICP values may

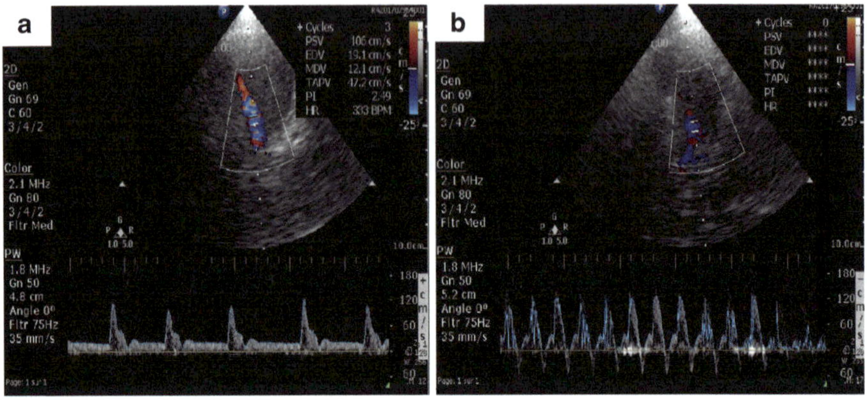

Fig. 1 Example of Transcranial Doppler in an adolescent with hepatic encephalopathy. Panel (**a**) displays a sharply defined systolic flow peak with low diastolic velocities, underlining the appearance of an intracranial pressure. Panel (**b**) displays a very sharp systolic peak retrograde flow during diastole highlighting a severe intracranial pressure and poor cerebral perfusion

impact disease progression and may help stabilize patients waiting for liver transplantation. Despite these potential benefits, many centers remain reluctant (including our center) to employ ICP monitors because of their inherent risks of bleeding in patients showing very abnormal coagulation. Recent studies have, however, shown that with appropriate coagulation control (which includes administration of Factor VII), the use of ICP monitoring is feasible, safe, associated with a low incidence of serious complications, and helps significantly in management. Its impact on patients' overall outcome has, however, to be proven [31, 32]. Conventional electroencephalography has been used in children with HE to screen for seizures, assess cerebral function, and predict outcome. In a small retrospective observational study of children and infants with ALF, children with a moderate or severely abnormal EEG were more likely to require liver transplant or die [33]. Spectral EEG analysis may help evaluate younger patients, allow quantitative and reproducible assessment of HE by non-neurologists in the intensive care unit [34]. Sensory evoked potentials are altered in patients with ALF. Small studies suggest their use in predicting those who may spontaneously recover from those who benefit from earlier liver transplant [35, 36].

Treatment

Management of HE depends on its severity (Fig. 2). All interventions and care are directed towards preventing the development of cerebral edema. General supportive measures of care in patients with severe HE include: (1) adequate systemic arterial blood pressure; (2) correction of electrolytes and glucose imbalances; (3) avoidance of hypoventilation; and (4) avoidance of hyperthermia. Adequate systemic arterial

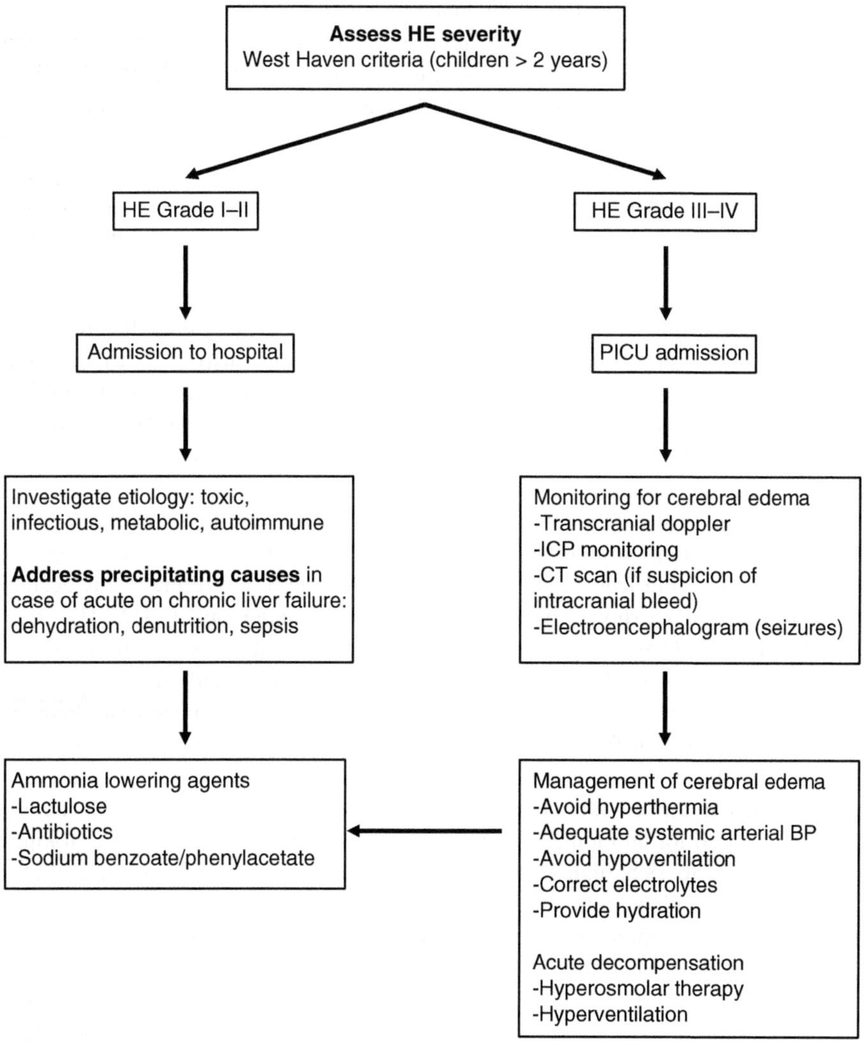

Fig. 2 Algorithm for the management of hepatic encephalopathy. BP blood pressure, CT computerized tomography, HE hepatic encephalopathy, ICP intracranial pressure monitoring, PICU pediatric intensive care unit

blood pressure, particularly in patients with impaired cerebral autoregulation, is of utmost importance. Elevated blood pressure can worsen intracranial hypertension, whereas low blood pressure can compromise cerebral blood flow. Adequate intravascular volume and vasopressors can be used to achieve normal blood pressure. ICP monitoring when installed can help titrate and guide management on an individual basis [32]. Head of bed should remain at 30 degrees to optimize cerebral venous drainage. Ventilator support needs to be cautiously titrated to avoid hypoventilation, which can cause cerebral vasodilation and worsen intracranial hypertension. Hyperventilation can help temporarily decrease ICP by causing cerebral vasoconstriction. However, it should be only used in context of acute rise in ICP as prolonged hyperventilation could potentially induce cerebral ischemia [37–40]. Furthermore, alkalosis favors the gaseous form and uptake of ammonia from the circulation to the BBB. Moderate hypothermia (32–33 °C) appears to be safe to treat patients with ICP unresponsive to mannitol [41, 42].

Pharmacologic management includes therapies guided to lower ammonia and those guided to lower intracranial hypertension. Lactulose reduces colonic pH and impairs the reuptake of glutamine in the intestine consequently lowering the production of ammonia [43]. Lactulose can be of use in patients with HE. However, it should be administered cautiously because overtreatment may result in significant electrolyte imbalances and dehydration. Antibiotics are also used to decrease ammonia, by lowering the production and absorption of gut-derived ammonia and reducing systemic inflammation [44]. Although N-acetylcystein has been shown to be potentially effective in adult non-acetaminophen induced ALF [45, 46], it has actually been shown to be detrimental in children [47]. Phenylacetate conjugates with glutamine to allow the renal excretion of ammonia. Sodium benzoate does the same by conjugating with glycine [48]. L-ornithine is a substrate of glutamine synthesis. A phase 2B efficacy and safety study of the role of Ornithine Phenylacetate in Hospitalized Cirrhotic patients with HE is underway (STOP-HE trial NCT01966419). Osmotic agents such as hypertonic saline or mannitol act by increasing blood osmolality, which causes an intracellular fluid shift towards the interstitial and intravascular space. This causes brain volume to decrease. Patients who receive mannitol for the management of cerebral edema are more likely to survive than those who do not receive it [49]. However, it should be used with caution and only in those with normal renal function. Continuous veno-venous hemofiltration is used for ammonia filtration and removal of proinflammatory cytokines [50]. Within 24 to 48 h, high volume hemofiltration decreases HE grade and allows better hemodynamic stability and overall may improve survival [50, 51]. In pediatrics, the proposed indications for initiation of therapy are high ammonia level (>200 μmol/L), hyponatremia, HE grade III or IV, fluid overload, and renal failure.

The supportive treatment in patients with severe HE includes adequate systemic arterial blood pressure, correction of electrolytes and glucose imbalances, normoventilation and normothermia, and lower ammonia blood level.

Outcome

Almost two-thirds of children diagnosed with ALF present or develop HE within 7 days of their initial symptoms. HE is an important marker of severity of disease. Indeed, up to 55% of children with severe HE (grades III or IV) and up to 26% of children with progressing HE will not survive their illness [18, 23]. Liver transplantation occurs more frequently in children who develop HE, have persistent mild HE, or with progressive HE. Younger age, diagnosis, HE, and liver function all influence prognosis.

Conclusion

Hepatic encephalopathy is a serious complication of acute liver failure, and when severe, a major cause of mortality in this population. Hyperammonemia, glutamine-induced astrocyte swelling, blood brain barrier disruption, cerebral dysregulation, and excitotoxicity are some of the many pathological processes involved in the development of HE and cerebral edema. Diagnosis of HE in young children can be difficult, as symptoms can be subtle, nonspecific, sometimes latent, and only visible at the terminal stages of liver failure. Complete reversal of HE ultimately depends on liver recovery or liver transplantation. Multiple surveillance and treatment modalities have, however, been developed to help prevent, detect, and control the progression of HE. In severe cases of HE with or without cerebral edema, ICP monitoring, hemofiltration, and ICP targeting treatments can help in managing and preventing progression of disease and help bridge recovery or liver transplantation. Transcranial Doppler is a noninvasive surveillance modality that can also help better understand each patient's individual cerebral physiology and better target treatment. When used with controlled coagulation, ICP monitoring can also help in managing severe cases of intracranial hypertension.

HE is a serious complication of acute liver failure. Further research to better understand the pathophysiology and development of HE is necessary to refine our management and improve long-term outcome.

References

1. Clemmesen JO, Larsen FS, Kondrup J, Hansen BA, Ott P. Cerebral herniation in patients with acute liver failure is correlated with arterial ammonia concentration. Hepatology. 1999;29(3):648–53.
2. Norenberg MD, Martinez-Hernandez A. Fine structural localization of glutamine synthetase in astrocytes of rat brain. Brain Res. 1979;161(2):303–10.
3. Skowronska M, Albrecht J. Alterations of blood brain barrier function in hyperammonemia: an overview. Neurotox Res. 2012;21(2):236–44.
4. Albrecht J, Norenberg MD. Glutamine: a Trojan horse in ammonia neurotoxicity. Hepatology. 2006;44(4):788–94.
5. Desjardins P, Du T, Jiang W, Peng L, Butterworth RF. Pathogenesis of hepatic encephalopathy and brain edema in acute liver failure: role of glutamine redefined. Neurochem Int. 2012;60(7):690–6.
6. Rama Rao KV, Jayakumar AR, Norenberg MD. Brain edema in acute liver failure: mechanisms and concepts. Metab Brain Dis. 2014;29(4):927–36.

7. Frontera JA. Metabolic encephalopathies in the critical care unit. Continuum (Minneap Minn). 2012;18(3):611–39.
8. Larsen FS, Gottstein J, Blei AT. Cerebral hyperemia and nitric oxide synthase in rats with ammonia-induced brain edema. J Hepatol. 2001;34(4):548–54.
9. Lockwood AH, Yap EW, Wong WH. Cerebral ammonia metabolism in patients with severe liver disease and minimal hepatic encephalopathy. J Cereb Blood Flow Metab. 1991;11(2):337–41.
10. Goldbecker A, Buchert R, Berding G, Bokemeyer M, Lichtinghagen R, Wilke F, et al. Blood-brain barrier permeability for ammonia in patients with different grades of liver fibrosis is not different from healthy controls. J Cereb Blood Flow Metab. 2010;30(7):1384–93.
11. Banks WA, Kastin AJ, Broadwell RD. Passage of cytokines across the blood-brain barrier. Neuroimmunomodulation. 1995;2(4):241–8.
12. Lockwood AH, Finn RD, Campbell JA, Richman TB. Factors that affect the uptake of ammonia by the brain: the blood-brain pH gradient. Brain Res. 1980;181(2):259–66.
13. Hermenegildo C, Monfort P, Felipo V. Activation of N-methyl-D-aspartate receptors in rat brain in vivo following acute ammonia intoxication: characterization by in vivo brain microdialysis. Hepatology. 2000;31(3):709–15.
14. Strauss G, Hansen BA, Kirkegaard P, Rasmussen A, Hjortrup A, Larsen FS. Liver function, cerebral blood flow autoregulation, and hepatic encephalopathy in fulminant hepatic failure. Hepatology. 1997;25(4):837–9.
15. Schliess F, Haussinger D. Hepatic encephalopathy and nitric oxide. J Hepatol. 2001;34(4):610–2.
16. Raghavan M, Marik PE. Therapy of intracranial hypertension in patients with fulminant hepatic failure. Neurocrit Care. 2006;4(2):179–89.
17. Wendon J, Lee W. Encephalopathy and cerebral edema in the setting of acute liver failure: pathogenesis and management. Neurocrit Care. 2008;9(1):97–102.
18. Squires RH Jr, Shneider BL, Bucuvalas J, Alonso E, Sokol RJ, Narkewicz MR, et al. Acute liver failure in children: the first 348 patients in the pediatric acute liver failure study group. J Pediatr. 2006;148(5):652–8.
19. Whittington PFAA. Fulminant hepatitis and acute liver failure. In: Kelly DA, editor. Disease of the lliver and biliary system in children. Oxford: Blackwell; 2003. p. 107.
20. Squires RH Jr. Acute liver failure in children. Semin Liver Dis. 2008;28(2):153–66.
21. Khungar V, Poordad F. Hepatic encephalopathy. Clin Liver Dis. 2012;16(2):301–20.
22. Cadranel JF, Lebiez E, Di Martino V, Bernard B, El Koury S, Tourbah A, et al. Focal neurological signs in hepatic encephalopathy in cirrhotic patients: an underestimated entity? Am J Gastroenterol. 2001;96(2):515–8.
23. Ng VL, Li R, Loomes KM, Leonis MA, Rudnick DA, Belle SH, et al. Outcomes of children with and without hepatic encephalopathy from the Pediatric Acute Liver Failure Study Group. J Pediatr Gastroenterol Nutr. 2016;63(3):357–64.
24. Toney NA, Bell MJ, Belle SH, Hardison RM, Rodriguez-Baez N, Loomes KM, et al. Hepatic encephalopathy in children with acute liver failure: utility of serum neuromarkers. J Pediatr Gastroenterol Nutr. 2019;69(1):108–15.
25. Suresh V, Aggarwal A. Optic nerve sheath diameter in children with acute liver failure and hepatic encephalopathy. Liver Int. 2020;41(1):233.
26. Dahaba AA, Worm HC, Zhu SM, Bao FP, Salah A, Zakaria S, et al. Sensitivity and specificity of bispectral index for classification of overt hepatic encephalopathy: a multicentre, observer blinded, validation study. Gut. 2008;57(1):77–83.
27. Munoz SJ. Difficult management problems in fulminant hepatic failure. Semin Liver Dis. 1993;13(4):395–413.
28. Aggarwal S, Obrist W, Yonas H, Kramer D, Kang Y, Scott V, et al. Cerebral hemodynamic and metabolic profiles in fulminant hepatic failure: relationship to outcome. Liver Transpl. 2005;11(11):1353–60.
29. Bellner J, Romner B, Reinstrup P, Kristiansson KA, Ryding E, Brandt L. Transcranial Doppler sonography pulsatility index (PI) reflects intracranial pressure (ICP). Surg Neurol. 2004;62(1):45–51; discussion.

30. Aggarwal S, Brooks DM, Kang Y, Linden PK, Patzer JF 2nd. Noninvasive monitoring of cerebral perfusion pressure in patients with acute liver failure using transcranial doppler ultrasonography. Liver Transpl. 2008;14(7):1048–57.
31. Rajajee V, Fontana RJ, Courey AJ, Patil PG. Protocol based invasive intracranial pressure monitoring in acute liver failure: feasibility, safety and impact on management. Crit Care. 2017;21(1):178.
32. Kamat P, Kunde S, Vos M, Vats A, Gupta N, Heffron T, et al. Invasive intracranial pressure monitoring is a useful adjunct in the management of severe hepatic encephalopathy associated with pediatric acute liver failure. Pediatr Crit Care Med. 2012;13(1):e33–8.
33. Hussain E, Grimason M, Goldstein J, Smith CM, Alonso E, Whitington PF, et al. EEG abnormalities are associated with increased risk of transplant or poor outcome in children with acute liver failure. J Pediatr Gastroenterol Nutr. 2014;58(4):449–56.
34. Press CA, Morgan L, Mills M, Stack CV, Goldstein JL, Alonso EM, et al. Spectral electroencephalogram analysis for the evaluation of encephalopathy grade in children with acute liver failure. Pediatr Crit Care Med. 2017;18(1):64–72.
35. Madl C, Grimm G, Ferenci P, Kramer L, Yeganehfar W, Oder W, et al. Serial recording of sensory evoked potentials: a noninvasive prognostic indicator in fulminant liver failure. Hepatology. 1994;20(6):1487–94.
36. Madl CKL, Gendo A. Prognostic accuracy of sensory evoked potentials (SEP) and arterial ammonia in predicting development of cerebral edema and death by cerebral herniation in patients with fulminant hepatic failure. Gastroenterology. 2000;118:1007A.
37. Bingaman WE, Frank JI. Malignant cerebral edema and intracranial hypertension. Neurol Clin. 1995;13(3):479–509.
38. Strauss G, Hansen BA, Knudsen GM, Larsen FS. Hyperventilation restores cerebral blood flow autoregulation in patients with acute liver failure. J Hepatol. 1998;28(2):199–203.
39. Ede R, Gimson AE, Cannalese J, Williams R. Cerebral oedema and monitoring of intracranial pressure in fulminant hepatic failure. Gastroenterol Jpn. 1982;17(2):163–76.
40. Ede RJ, Gimson AE, Bihari D, Williams R. Controlled hyperventilation in the prevention of cerebral oedema in fulminant hepatic failure. J Hepatol. 1986;2(1):43–51.
41. Jalan R, Rose C. Hypothermia in acute liver failure. Metab Brain Dis. 2004;19(3–4):215–21.
42. Karvellas CJ, Todd Stravitz R, Battenhouse H, Lee WM, Schilsky ML, Group USALFS. Therapeutic hypothermia in acute liver failure: a multicenter retrospective cohort analysis. Liver Transpl. 2015;21(1):4–12.
43. Hadjihambi A, Khetan V, Jalan R. Pharmacotherapy for hyperammonemia. Expert Opin Pharmacother. 2014;15(12):1685–95.
44. Furue M, Seki Y, Oohara K, Ishibashi Y. Basal cell epithelioma arising in a patient with Hailey-Hailey's disease. Int J Dermatol. 1987;26(7):461–2.
45. Blei AT, Cordoba J. Practice Parameters Committee of the American College of G. Hepatic Encephalopathy. Am J Gastroenterol. 2001;96(7):1968–76.
46. Furuta I. Selection of bedside tests. Bacteriologic tests. Rinsho Byori. 1987;Spec No 72:52–9.
47. Squires RH, Dhawan A, Alonso E, Narkewicz MR, Shneider BL, Rodriguez-Baez N, et al. Intravenous N-acetylcysteine in pediatric patients with nonacetaminophen acute liver failure: a placebo-controlled clinical trial. Hepatology. 2013;57(4):1542–9.
48. Sushma S, Dasarathy S, Tandon RK, Jain S, Gupta S, Bhist MS. Sodium benzoate in the treatment of acute hepatic encephalopathy: a double-blind randomized trial. Hepatology. 1992;16(1):138–44.
49. Canalese J, Gimson AE, Davis C, Mellon PJ, Davis M, Williams R. Controlled trial of dexamethasone and mannitol for the cerebral oedema of fulminant hepatic failure. Gut. 1982;23(7):625–9.
50. Chevret L, Durand P, Lambert J, Essouri S, Balu L, Devictor D, et al. High-volume hemofiltration in children with acute liver failure*. Pediatr Crit Care Med. 2014;15(7):e300–5.
51. Jalan R. Pathophysiological basis of therapy of raised intracranial pressure in acute liver failure. Neurochem Int. 2005;47(1–2):78–83.

Liver Failure and the Kidneys

Jean-Philippe Roy

Introduction

Acute kidney injuries (AKI) are common in acutely ill children admitted in pediatric intensive care units (PICU) and occur in approximately 1 out of 4 patients [1]. Children with acute liver failure (ALF) or acute on chronic liver failure (ACLF) are a particularly complex population and are at increased risk of diverse complications and organs failure, including kidney dysfunction [2]. While AKI can result from the same usual culprits, nephrotoxic medications and sepsis being among the most frequent, those patients are also at risk of decreased kidney function in the setting of hepatorenal syndrome (HRS) [3–5]. This condition is characterized by lower renal function with decreased renal blood flow that is unresponsive to fluid expansion and is associated with increased morbidity and mortality [6, 7]. In adults, AKI have been reported to occur in about half of patients with cirrhotic liver disease after the first few years of their onset of ascites. Of those, around 8% were attributable to HRS [8]. In children, the incidence of HRS is not well defined as there is no recent study evaluating that aspect based on more current definitions of HRS. Older studies using the adult definition of HRS at the time estimated an average of 5% of HRS in children with chronic liver disease (CLD), before their liver transplantation. However, this would probably underreport HRS by current criteria, better suited for diagnosing altered renal function in children [7, 9]. HRS can develop gradually in a patient with a long-standing cirrhotic liver disease but tends to occur more frequently in decompensated states. Infections (e.g. spontaneous bacterial peritonitis) and variceal bleedings are among the most common precipitating factors while advanced portal hypertension with ascites and hyponatremia are chief risk factors [6, 7].

J.-P. Roy (✉)
Nephrology Unit, Department of Pediatrics, CHU Sainte-Justine, University of Montreal, Montreal, QC, Canada
e-mail: jean-philippe.roy.1@umontreal.ca

P. Jouvet, F. Alvarez (eds.), *Liver Diseases in the Pediatric Intensive Care Unit*,
https://doi.org/10.1007/978-3-030-79132-2_5

These elements together make HRS more common in ACLF or acutely ill patients with CLD, although it still can occur in ALF.

Physiopathology

The occurrence of renal dysfunction in the setting of HRS is the result of multiple factors. Initially thought to be mainly caused by decreased renal perfusion, current models of its pathogenesis now point at circulatory dysfunction combined with evidence of systemic inflammation [7, 10]. Those mechanisms, studied in adult patients, are believed to be applicable to children with liver diseases, but few studies explore the pathogenesis of HRS itself at the pediatric age.

Circulatory dysfunction involves multiples anomalies, the most central of which being splanchnic vasodilation. As cirrhotic liver disease progresses, the increased resistance in intrahepatic vascular flow that characterizes portal hypertension leads to the release of vasodilating mediators in splanchnic arteries. In turn, the vasodilation of the splanchnic bed leads to a systemic hypotension and general lower peripheral vascular resistance [11]. Nitric oxide, glucagon, carbon monoxide, prostacyclin, and other molecules are generally held as the main mediators of splanchnic vasodilation [7]. Decrease in peripheral vascular resistance leads to a cardiac compensation by a hyperdynamic state and renal hypoperfusion. Those then trigger a physiological response involving renin angiotensin aldosterone system (RAAS), the sympathetic nervous system and non-osmotic vasopressin secretion. These mechanisms work in concert to promote sodium and water retention as an attempt to correct the perceived pathological state (cardiac underfilling and decreased renal blood flow), but since splanchnic vasodilation persists, they lead to ascites formation without improving renal hypoperfusion [7, 10, 11].

While renal vasoconstriction is central in HRS, patients with more severe phenotypes of kidney, or other organs, dysfunction in the setting of HRS were exhibiting greater systemic inflammation activation. Moreover, patients with CLD with higher biomarkers of inflammation at a stable state of cirrhosis were at greater risk of ACLF and death during an episode of liver decompensation [12]. Bacterial translocation and bacterial peritonitis being triggers for HRS in predisposed patients, those events worsen renal dysfunction even in the absence of septic shock. Endotoxins and bacterial DNA, considered pathogen-associated molecular patterns (PAMPs), play an important role in inflammatory upregulation. Cytokines released by monocytes once activated by PAMPs (i.e. Tumor necrosis factor alpha, interleukin 6, and interleukin 1 beta) have been associated with renal dysfunction in ALF and ACLF [13–15]. Tissue injury caused by PAMPs and inflammation will in turn activate damage-associated molecular patterns (DAMPs) that increase the inflammatory response. Those patterns can lead to a worsening glomerular filtration rate (GFR) in an already hypoperfused kidney.

Children with chronic liver disease show progression of portal hypertension, which contribute to renal hypoperfusion and systemic inflammation, thus increasing their susceptibility for developing hepatorenal syndrome.

Many elements support that HRS is predominantly functional; (1) few to no histological changes are seen in kidneys during autopsies of patients with this condition, (2) renal dysfunction is improved by vasoconstrictors, (3) it is commonly reversible after liver transplantation and (4) kidneys of patients in HRS can be viably used for renal transplantation [10, 16]. However, biomarkers of kidney tissue damage are not entirely negative in patients with HRS, as it would be expected from a purely functional renal dysfunction. Urine neutrophil gelatinase-associated lipocaline (NGAL) is extensively studied as a biomarker of kidney damage, distinguishing functional decrease in glomerular filtration rate (GFR) from intrinsic kidney damage like acute tubular necrosis (ATN). When studied in hospitalized CLD patients with AKI, urine NGAL was significantly higher in ATN compared to HRS. However, levels could still be elevated to a lesser extent in HRS and higher levels still had prognostic value in those patients [17]. Those evidences would support some level of kidney damage, possibly associated with inflammation in the setting of PAMPs and DAMPs, coinciding with the characteristic severe renal vasoconstriction and decreased blood flow.

Two main different clinical phenotypes of HRS are seen, one with an acute onset of decrease in renal function happening over a few days (formerly called type 1) and which generally have an infectious trigger, and one with a more chronic onset that evolves over weeks (formerly called type 2) that tends to be characterized by a progressive diuretic-resistant ascites. The degree of contribution of those different pathologic mechanisms together may be responsible for the clinical phenotype [6, 7, 10].

Hepatorenal syndrome is predominantly functional with renal vasoconstriction due to splanchnic vasodilation and worsened by inflammation.

Definition and Diagnosis

The definition of HRS by the International Club of Ascites (ICA) underwent many changes over the years, especially the serum creatinine (SCr) criteria. Initially using a fixed cut-off of 1.5 mg/dL (133 µmol/L), this proved to be clinically inadequate for the interindividual variability in SCr levels. This commonly used biomarker of glomerular filtration produced by muscle and protein metabolism varies greatly depending on age, size, and muscle mass among other clinical factors. Thus, using a fixed cut-off to define a significant reduction in GFR not only underdiagnoses HRS in children, elderly people, and malnourished or muscle-wasted individuals but also creates clinical confusion in patients with preexisting chronic kidney disease (CKD). The initial definition also included a delay criteria of 2 weeks for SCr to double from its baseline to diagnose an acute form of HRS. This was thought to postpone the initiation of vasopressor treatments and could potentially be deleterious since a higher level of SCr at the introduction of those therapies is associated with worst outcome. To make those criteria more clinically accurate and to harmonize the definition of this type of kidney impairment with already existing and broadly accepted definitions of AKI and CKD (from Kidney Disease: Improving Global Outcome (KDIGO)), the ICA revised HRS definition in 2015 and now uses the term HRS-AKI [6, 10, 18]. This HRS-AKI definition correlates well with worst outcome in patients with cirrhosis [19, 20].

Given their physiology and frequent low urine output in cirrhotic patients, concerns were raised regarding the use of KDIGO urine output (UO) criteria for defining HRS-AKI. While excluded from their revision in 2015, the importance of AKI-UO criteria is now emerging as it not only increases AKI diagnosis accuracy, but it is also associated with increased mortality in patients with CLD, even in the absence of AKI by SCr definition [21]. More recently, the European Association for the Study of the Liver (EASL) and other authors suggested that UO criteria be used to define AKI and potentially HRS-AKI in patients with CLD when reliably assessed using a urinary catheter [10, 22]. They also suggested that the formerly called type 2 HRS, now referred to as HRS-non-AKI, be classified either as HRS-CKD, when renal dysfunction is present for more than 3 months without SCr returning to its baseline, or as HRS-acute kidney disease (AKD) in patients with prolonged SCr rise for less than 3 months [10, 22]. Given the occurrence of HRS in acutely decompensated CLD patients and severe ALF, authors have also suggested that those clinical scenarios be included in the diagnostic criteria, instead of the previous requirement of cirrhotic disease with ascites at baseline [10].

To diagnose HRS-AKI as the cause of a new renal dysfunction, a patient must have a significant liver disease (cirrhosis with ascites, ALF, or ACLF) and the kidney impairment must meet AKI criteria (see Table 1). Other causes of AKI must not be present, like shock or nephrotoxic drugs exposure (i.e. nonsteroid anti-inflammatory drugs, aminoglycoside, vancomycin, contrast agents, etc.), and there must be no signs of structural kidney injury or disease (macroscopic hematuria or microscopic >50 red blood cell per high power field, proteinuria above 500 mg per day, or abnormalities on kidney ultrasound) unless those are attributable to a preexisting known renal condition. To ensure that kidney impairment is not caused by intravascular depletion and low oncotic pressure, it must also be unresponsive to intravascular fluid expansion (no diuretic and 25% albumin infusion for at least 2 days) (see Table 1 for full criteria details) [10, 18, 22]. In critically ill patients, especially in the context of an infection (i.e. sepsis, spontaneous bacterial peritonitis), clinicians must use their judgment when assessing the etiology of renal dysfunction. Many infectious processes, or drugs used to treat them, can induce AKI including ATN or tubular dysfunction. However, those events can also trigger a spiral leading to HRS-AKI in a predisposed patient, by induction of systemic inflammation through PAMPs and DAMPs. When a significant infectious or toxic cause is thought to be responsible for AKI, close monitoring is needed to assess if an improvement in kidney function is observed. When kidney function fails to improve or worsen despite treating the initial causes (i.e. supporting shock, antibiotics, withdrawal of nephrotoxic agents, etc.) then HRS-AKI is reconsidered.

Table 1 Diagnostic criteria and classification for hepatorenal syndrome

Diagnostic criteria				
Cirrhosis with ascitis (or ALF/ACLF)[a]				
AKI by SCr criteria below (or UO criteria below)[a,b]				
Absence of shock				
No current or recent use of nephrotoxic drugs				
No response or only partial response to at least 2 days of diuretic withdrawal and volume expansion with 25% albumin (1 g/kg/day, up to 100 g/day)				
Absence of parenchymal renal disease,[c] defined as: Proteinuria > 500 mg/day Macroscopic hematuria or microscopic >50 RBC/HPF Abnormal renal ultrasound				
HRS subtypes classification				
Previous classification	Current classification		Criteria	
Type 1	HRS-AKI	Stage 1	SCr:	1.5–1.9 times increase or >0.3 mg/dL (26.5 μmol/L) from baseline within 48 h
			UO:	<0.5 mL/kg/h × 6–12 h[a,b]
		Stage 2	SCr:	2.0–2.9 times increase from baseline
			UO:	<0.5 mL/kg/h × >12 h[a,b]
		Stage 3	SCr:	>3.0 times increase from baseline or >4 mg/dL (353.6 μmol/L) or initiation of renal replacement therapy or GFR < 35 mL/min/1.73 m^2 in patients between 2 and 18 y/o
			UO:	<0.5 mL/kg/h × 24 h or anuria × >12 h[a,b]
Type 2	HRS-non-AKI			
	HRS-AKD		GFR < 60 mL/min/1.73 m^2 for <3 months without other structural causes (in patients between 2 and 18 y/o, a cut-off <90 mL/min/1.73 m^2 is advisable)[d]	
			Persistent SCr increase of >50% of from baseline for <3 months	
	HRS-CKD		GFR < 60 mL/min/1.73 m^2 for <3 months without other structural causes (in patients between 2 and 18 y/o, a cut-off <90 mL/min/1.73 m^2 is advisable)[d]	

ACLF acute on chronic liver failure, *AKD* acute kidney disease, *ALF* acute liver failure, *CKD* chronic kidney disease, *EASL* European Society for the Study of the Liver, *GFR* glomerular filtration rate, *HPF* high power field, *HRS* hepatorenal syndrome, *ICA* International Club of Ascites, *RBC* red blood cell, *SCr* serum creatinine, *UO* urine output, *y/o* year old

[a]EASL suggested addition to the ICA 2015 guidelines

[b]This parameter requires a urinary catheter to be used

[c]Excluding knowing preexisting conditions (i.e. glomerulonephritis, diabetic nephropathy)

[d]Children and adolescents have normal GFR usually around 100–120 mL/min/1.73 m^2

AKI by SCr KDIGO criteria is defined by its elevation from patients' baseline. An increase of 1.5–1.9 times from baseline (or an absolute rise of ≥0.3 mg/dL or 26.5 μmol/L) within 48 h is defined as a stage 1 AKI, 2.0–2.9 times increase for stage 2, and more than 3.0 times increase for stage 3 [23]. Many patients are admitted to the hospital with preexisting renal dysfunction, making SCr on admission unreliable for establishing a patient's baseline. Moreover, since baseline SCr can change over time (e.g. normal increase over time in children, gradual muscle wasting in chronically ill patient) it is recommended to use the lowest level of SCr available in the preceding last 3 months [10]. For acutely ill children older than 2 years of age who have never had a previous measurement of SCr level, a baseline can be derived by inverse calculation of the Schwartz formula, normally used to estimate GFR, if normal kidney function can be assumed prior to current episode (see Eq. 1) [24]. Baselines obtained by this method are conservative and can slightly underestimate true baselines in some children.

Equation 1: Reversed revised 2009 bedside Schwartz formula

$$\begin{aligned} &\text{Estimated SCr baseline}\left(\text{mg / dL}\right) \\ &= 0.413 \times \left(\text{Height}\left(\text{cm}\right) / 120\left(\text{ml / min/ 1.73 m}^2\right)\right) \\ &\text{Estimated SCr baseline}\left(\mu\text{mol / L}\right) \\ &= 36.517 \times \left(\text{Height}\left(\text{cm}\right) / 120\left(\text{ml / min/ 1.73 m}^2\right)\right) \end{aligned} \tag{1}$$

> The diagnosis of hepatorenal syndrome includes a significant liver disease and the kidney impairment must meet AKI criteria (see Table 1) without intravascular depletion and low oncotic pressure.

Management

When renal dysfunction is diagnosed in a critically ill child with liver disease, close monitoring of their renal function and investigation of AKI differential diagnosis should be initiated. In accordance with KDIGO and ICA recommendations, as early as stage 1, the following three measures are required: (1) nephrotoxic drugs should be removed as much as possible, signs or history of hypovolemia should be corrected with a trial of intravascular expansion and diuretic withdrawal, (2) potential infections should be carefully sought with early initiation of antibiotics if there is sufficient clinical suspicion, and (3) hemodynamic status should be assessed and supported if needed.

The use of over-the-counter medications should also be questioned for possible nephrotoxic exposure (i.e. nonsteroidal anti-inflammatory drugs). While there is controversial data on the role of beta-blockers and vasodilators in cirrhotic patients with renal dysfunction, 2015 ICA guidelines recommend withdrawing those in AKI [18, 25]. In patients in whom stage 1 AKI progresses despite these interventions, or who initially present with stage 2 or 3, a formal volume expansion trial should be performed with 1 g/kg/day of 25% albumin infusion (up to 100 g/day) and diuretic withdrawal (if not already done) for at least 2 days. If there is a complete renal function recovery with these measures i.e. normalization of SCr within 0.3 mg/dL (26.5 μmol/L) of the patient's baseline, HRS-AKI is ruled out and SCr should be followed closely (every 2 to 4 days during the hospital stay and every 2 to 4 weeks for 6 months following discharge) [18]. If a stage 2 or 3 AKI persists or progresses in patients fulfilling HRS-AKI diagnostic criteria (see Table 1), this diagnosis is then ruled in and vasoconstrictors with albumin infusions must be initiated. There is no specific recommendation for patients with persistent stage 1 AKI who do not progress after initial support. Given the heterogeneity of this group, each condition must be assessed and treated on a case-by-case basis. In the 2015 ICA recommendations, all experts agreed that patients in this specific group should be treated with vasoconstrictors and albumin if they have a SCr level above 1.5 mg/dL (133 μmol/L), based on the previous HRS definition. However, this is not applicable to children, since their baseline SCr is lower and a fixed SCr value is not an adequate decision threshold [18]. (see Fig. 1 for management algorithm).

Vasoconstrictors (i.e. terlipressine, noradrenaline, and the combination of midodrine and octreotide) are used in HRS to counteract splanchnic arterial vasodilation and break the vicious cycle that perpetuates renal hypoperfusion. Several randomized controlled trials (RCT) and meta-analyses have shown that these treatments, in combination with albumin infusions, improve renal function and survival in adult patients with type 1 HRS [6, 7, 18, 22]. Given the lower incidence of HRS in children, as well as the inadequacy of its previous definition for a pediatric population, RCT were impractical or impossible. There is currently little or no evidence, particularly in children, evaluating their response and prognosis with vasoconstrictor therapies for HRS treatment. Nevertheless, these vasoconstrictors are used in children with HRS-AKI based on adult studies and data from other applications of those drugs [4, 26, 27]. The previous definition of type 1 HRS used a higher SCr threshold. Therefore, since it has also been observed that a higher SCr value at vasoconstrictor treatment initiation is an independent risk factor of a lower response rate, these therapies are expected to be at least as effective with the new HRS-AKI definition. However, this assumption needs to be studied [10, 18]. A meta-analysis found no statistical difference between terlipressine, noradrenaline, and midodrine with octreotide in the improvement of survival, but there was a potential superiority of terlipressine in HRS reversal over midodrine with octreotide. A second meta-analysis suggested that terlipressine was superior to noradrenaline in reversing HRS, and midodrine with octreotide was inferior to both [28, 29]. However, terlipressine is expensive and not readily available in all countries, while noradrenaline needs a central venous line and PICU admission for monitoring. Given the nature of those drugs, patients have to be monitored for side effects including hypertension, peripheral and intestinal ischemia, diarrhea, and angina pectoris. However, some increase in blood pressure should be expected. If SCr does not improve by more than 25% after 2-3 days, it could indicate underdosing and the need for increased

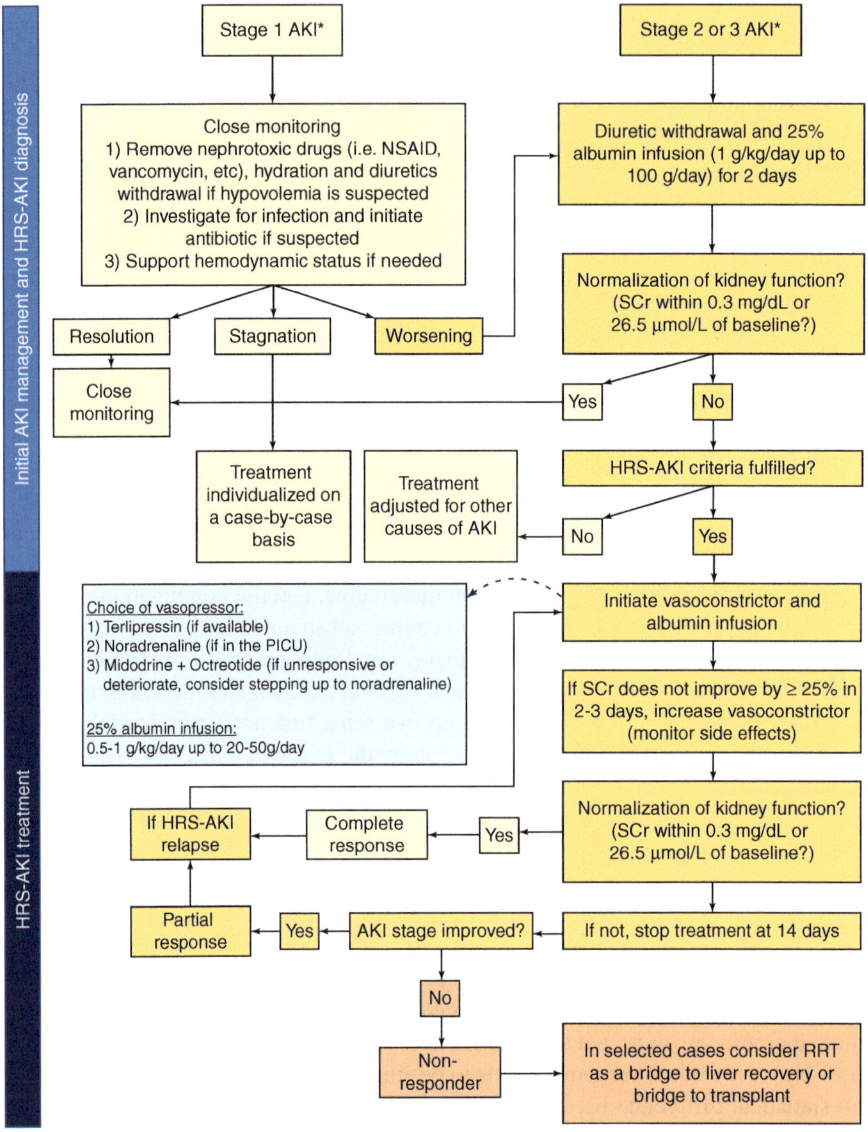

Fig. 1 HRS-AKI diagnosis and management. HRS hepatorenal syndrome, AKI acute kidney injury, NSAID nonsteroidal anti-inflammatory drugs, PICU pediatric intensive care unit, SCr serum creatinine, RRT renal replacement therapy. *AKI by KDIGO criteria, see Table 1. (Figure partially inspired from the International Club of Ascites 2015 guidelines)

vasoconstrictor administration. Vasoconstrictor doses should then be gradually increased with careful monitoring of tolerance and side effects [6, 10, 22]. Albumin infusion dosage varies according to studies, generally 20 to 40 g/day in adults, but recommendations of 25 to 50 g/day can also be found for use with vasoconstrictors,

0.5–1.0 g/kg/day is usually administered in children [10, 18, 22]. There is no threshold of serum albumin at which HRS-AKI is known to be more responsive to vasoconstrictor. It is, however, reasonable to aim for serum levels above 20–25 g/L when administering daily infusions in combination with a vasoconstrictor in children with HRS-AKI. Vasoconstrictors and albumin should be stopped in case of a complete response or after 14 days. An improvement of SCr within 0.3 mg/dL (26.5 μmol/L) of baseline is classified as a complete response, a persistent AKI with an improved stage is considered a partial response, while a failure to improve after 14 days corresponds to a nonresponder. Failure to respond to vasoconstrictor and albumin is associated with worst outcome and increased mortality [10, 22]. In responders, up to 20% of HRS will relapse after the discontinuation of those therapies. Re-treating is usually effective but may require multiple courses over an extended period of time depending on the underlying liver condition [10, 22]. Vasoconstrictors are effective to improve renal function in HRS-non-AKI. However, relapses after discontinuation are frequent and are not associated with outcome improvement, either pre- or post-transplantation. For those reasons, vasoconstrictors are currently not recommended in HRS-non-AKI [7, 10, 22, 30, 31].

Unless the underlying liver disease is expected to be transient or to significantly improve, liver transplantation remains the treatment of choice in HRS[31, 32].

Some patients with HRS-AKI may qualify for extracorporeal therapies, including continuous renal replacement therapy. Standard dialysis indications are usually used which, in children, often include fluid overload [33]. Nevertheless, those therapies must be considered only as bridge to liver improvement or to liver transplantation, and some patients may not qualify for it in this context [22].

Transjugular intrahepatic portosystemic shunt (TIPS) has been studied mostly in adults with type 2 HRS (now called HRS-non-AKI) and has shown some benefits, including renal function improvement. However, it is rarely used in practice because of the advanced stage of liver disease and the high risk of hepatic encephalopathy [6, 7, 22, 34].

Conclusion

AKI on its own increases morbidity and mortality in acutely ill children, death being significantly increased from 2.5% to 11% in children with severe AKI (stage 2 or 3) in PICU, regardless of dialysis need [1]. In the context of decompensated liver disease, severe AKI carries an even worse prognosis with mortality up to 50% in patients with HRS-AKI stage 2–3 [35]. In adult RCT on vasoconstrictor therapy for HRS-AKI, mortality is often 40–90% without liver transplant [6].

Early recognition and treatment of HRS-AKI through optimizing supportive measures is believed to be central in reversing renal dysfunction, especially in acutely ill patients, to improve survival chances until liver recovery or transplant is achieved.

References

1. Kaddourah A, Basu RK, Bagshaw SM, Goldstein SL. Epidemiology of acute kidney injury in critically ill children and young adults. N Engl J Med. 2017;376:11–20.
2. Devictor D, Tissieres P, Afanetti M, Debray D. Acute liver failure in children. Clin Res Hepatol Gastroenterol. 2011;35:430–7.
3. Sutherland SM, Kwiatkowski DM. Acute kidney injury in children. Adv Chronic Kidney Dis. 2017;24:253–63. https://doi.org/10.1053/j.ackd.2017.09.007.
4. Deep A, Saxena R, Jose B. Acute kidney injury in children with chronic liver disease. Pediatr Nephrol. 2019;34:45–59.
5. Goldstein SL. Medication-induced acute kidney injury. Curr Opin Crit Care. 2016;22:542–5.
6. Francoz C, Durand F, Kahn JA, Genyk YS, Nadim MK. Hepatorenal syndrome. Clin J Am Soc Nephrol. 2019;14:774–81.
7. Liu PMF, de Carvalho ST, Fradico PF, Cazumbá MLB, Campos RGB, Simões e Silva AC. Hepatorenal syndrome in children: a review. Pediatr Nephrol. 2020. https://doi.org/10.1007/s00467-020-04762-6.
8. Montoliu S, Ballesté B, Planas R, Álvarez MA, Rivera M, Miquel M, et al. Incidence and prognosis of different types of functional renal failure in cirrhotic patients with ascites. Clin Gastroenterol Hepatol. 2010;8:616–22.
9. Ellis D, Avner ED, Starzl TE. Renal failure in children with hepatic failure undergoing liver transplantation. J Pediatr. 1986;108:393–8.
10. Angeli P, Garcia-Tsao G, Nadim MK, Parikh CR. News in pathophysiology, definition and classification of hepatorenal syndrome: a step beyond the International Club of Ascites (ICA) consensus document. J Hepatol. 2019;71:811–22.
11. Moore CM, Van Thiel DH. Cirrhotic ascites review: pathophysiology, diagnosis and management. World J Hepatol. 2013;5:251–63.
12. Trebicka J, Amoros A, Pitarch C, Titos E, Alcaraz-Quiles J, Schierwagen R, et al. Addressing profiles of systemic inflammation across the different clinical phenotypes of acutely decompensated cirrhosis. Front Immunol. 2019;10:476. https://doi.org/10.3389/fimmu.2019.00476.
13. Navasa M, Follo A, Filella X, Jiménez W, Francitorra A, Planas R, et al. Tumor necrosis factor and interleukin-6 in spontaneous bacterial peritonitis in cirrhosis: relationship with the development of renal impairment and mortality. Hepatology. 1998;27:1227–32.
14. Wiest R, Lawson M, Geuking M. Pathological bacterial translocation in liver cirrhosis. J Hepatol. 2014;60:197–209.
15. Moreau R, Jalan R, Gines P, Pavesi M, Angeli P, Cordoba J, et al. Acute-on-chronic liver failure is a distinct syndrome that develops in patients with acute decompensation of cirrhosis. Gastroenterology. 2013;144:1426–1437.e9.
16. Koppel MH, Coburn JW, Mims MM, Goldstein H, Boyle JD, Rubini ME. Transplantation of cadaveric kidneys from patients with hepatorenal syndrome. Evidence for the functional nature of renal failure in advanced liver disease. N Engl J Med. 1969;280:1367–71.
17. Huelin P, Solà E, Elia C, Solé C, Risso A, Moreira R, et al. Neutrophil gelatinase-associated Lipocalin for assessment of acute kidney injury in cirrhosis: a prospective study. Hepatology. 2019;70:319–33.
18. Angeli P, Ginès P, Wong F, Bernardi M, Boyer TD, Gerbes A, et al. Diagnosis and management of acute kidney injury in patients with cirrhosis: revised consensus recommendations of the International Club of Ascites. J Hepatol. 2015;62:968–74.
19. Piano S, Rosi S, Maresio G, Fasolato S, Cavallin M, Romano A, et al. Evaluation of the acute kidney injury network criteria in hospitalized patients with cirrhosis and ascites. J Hepatol. 2013;59:482–9.
20. Fagundes C, Barreto R, Guevara M, Garcia E, Solà E, Rodríguez E, et al. A modified acute kidney injury classification for diagnosis and risk stratification of impairment of kidney function in cirrhosis. J Hepatol. 2013;59:474–81.

21. Amathieu R, Al-Khafaji A, Sileanu FE, Foldes E, DeSensi R, Hilmi I, et al. Significance of oliguria in critically ill patients with chronic liver disease. Hepatology. 2017;66:1592–600.
22. Angeli P, Bernardi M, Villanueva C, Francoz C, Mookerjee RP, Trebicka J, et al. EASL clinical practice guidelines for the management of patients with decompensated cirrhosis. J Hepatol. 2018;69:406–60.
23. Khwaja A. KDIGO clinical practice guidelines for acute kidney injury. Nephron – Clin Pract. 2012;120:179–84.
24. Zappitelli M, Joseph L, Gupta IR, Bell L, Paradis G. Validation of child serum creatinine-based prediction equations for glomerular filtration rate. Pediatr Nephrol. 2007;22:272–81.
25. Kidney Disease: Improving Global Outcome (KDIGO) Acute Kidney Injury Work Group. KDIGO clinical practice guidelines for acute kidney injury. Kidney Int Suppl. 2012;2:138.
26. Saxena R, Anand A, Deep A. Use of terlipressin in critically ill children with liver disease. BMC Nephrol. 2020;21:1–6.
27. Debray D, Yousef N, Durand P. New management options for end-stage chronic liver disease and acute liver failure: potential for pediatric patients. Pediatr Drugs. 2006;8:1–13.
28. Israelsen M, Krag A, Gluud LL. Terlipressin versus other vasoactive drugs for hepatorenal syndrome. Cochrane Database Syst Rev. 2017; 2017. https://doi.org/10.1002/14651858.CD011532.
29. Wang L, Long Y, Li KX, Xu GS. Pharmacological treatment of hepatorenal syndrome: a network meta-analysis. Gastroenterol Rep. 2020;8:111–8.
30. Rodriguez E, Henrique Pereira G, Solà E, Elia C, Barreto R, Pose E, et al. Treatment of type 2 hepatorenal syndrome in patients awaiting transplantation: effects on kidney function and transplantation outcomes. Liver Transpl. 2015;21:1347–54.
31. Restuccia T, Ortega R, Guevara M, Ginès P, Alessandria C, Ozdogan O, et al. Effects of treatment of hepatorenal syndrome before transplantation on posttransplantation outcome. A case-control study. J Hepatol. 2004;40:140–6.
32. McDiarmid SV. Renal function in pediatric liver transplant patients. Kidney Int Suppl. 1996;53:S77–84.
33. Symons JM, Chua AN, Somers MJG, Baum MA, Bunchman TE, Benfield MR, et al. Demographic characteristics of pediatric continuous renal replacement therapy: a report of the prospective pediatric continuous renal replacement therapy registry. Clin J Am Soc Nephrol. 2007;2:732–8.
34. Charilaou P, Devani K, Petrosyan R, Reddy C, Pyrsopoulos N. Inpatient mortality benefit with transjugular intrahepatic portosystemic shunt for hospitalized hepatorenal syndrome patients. Dig Dis Sci. 2020;65:3378–88.
35. Lal BB, Alam S, Sood V, Rawat D, Khanna R. Profile, risk factors and outcome of acute kidney injury in paediatric acute-on-chronic liver failure. Liver Int. 2018;38:1777–84.

Liver Failure and Extracorporeal Therapies

Lucile Barcat, Jean-Philippe Roy, and Philippe Jouvet

Acute liver failure (ALF) occurs in 17 cases per 100,000 per year in the United States. Due to lack of data, the incidence in the pediatric population, as well as its mortality, is not well defined [1–3].

The management of severe acute liver failure (ALF) or acute-on-chronic liver failure (ACLF) admitted in intensive care unit (ICU) aims to maintain hemodynamic and respiratory status, avoid bleeding and prevent infections in order to prevent progression to multiorgan failure [1, 4]. In severe acute renal failure, whatever the cause (see chapter on Liver Failure and the Kidneys), renal replacement therapy (RRT) can be indicated. RRT removes only small molecular weight soluble toxins, and several other extracorporeal liver support therapies (ELST) are proposed to address liver detoxification and/or protein synthesis dysfunction [3, 5–8]. This chapter details current knowledge on ELST for the management of critically ill children with ALF.

L. Barcat (✉)
Pediatric Intensive Care Unit, Department of Pediatrics, CHU Sainte-Justine, Université de Montréal, Montreal, QC, Canada

J.-P. Roy
Nephrology Unit, Department of Pediatrics, CHU Sainte-Justine, University of Montreal, Montreal, QC, Canada
e-mail: jean-philippe.roy.1@umontreal.ca

P. Jouvet
Pediatric Intensive Care Unit - Department of Pediatrics of Sainte Justine Hospital, University of Montreal, Montréal, QC, Canada
e-mail: philippe.jouvet.med@ssss.gouv.qc.ca

P. Jouvet, F. Alvarez (eds.), *Liver Diseases in the Pediatric Intensive Care Unit*, https://doi.org/10.1007/978-3-030-79132-2_6

Renal Replacement Therapies

Peritoneal dialysis (PD), intermittent hemodialysis (iHD), and continuous renal replacement therapy (CRRT) are the different methods of RRT. They can be effective at removing ammonia, one of the toxin metabolites in ALF. Ammonia is a small soluble molecule (molecular mass 17 g/mol) that does not significantly bind to albumin or other proteins, thus dialysis is effective for its removal. However, RRT is ineffective at removing highly protein-bound toxins and those with molecular weight above 50–60 kDa, leaving a large part of ALF toxins undialyzed. Institutional preference, local technical skills, and methods availability on site determine the choice of dialysis modality depending on clinical scenarios. iHD and CRRT are more effective than PD at clearing toxins. If fluid overload correction is required, CRRT offer a greater hemodynamic stability than iHD by allowing a slower ultrafiltration rate on a longer period of time. The final choice of modality should be a multidisciplinary decision including critical care teams, nephrologist, hepatologist, and metabolism team [9, 10].

The RRT indication in case of acute renal failure is detailed in the chapter on kidney failure. For the management of liver failure, the indication is mainly based, but not only, on ammonia blood level. Recent consensus guidelines for the management of hyperammonemia were published in 2020 [9]. While they are mostly dedicated to inborn errors of metabolism with isolated hyperammonemia as opposed to a more mixed and complex toxins accumulation in ALF, there is a rational for using those recommendations as guidance on the indications for RRT in ALF but clinicians need to personalize their decision since ALF literature was not included. The criteria for RRT indication are one of the following four:

- Rapidly deteriorating neurological status, coma, or cerebral edema with blood ammonia level >150 μmol/L
- Presence of moderate-to-severe encephalopathy
- Persistently high serum ammonia levels >400 μmol/L refractory to medical treatment
- Rapid rise in ammonia levels >300 μmol/L within few hours that cannot be controlled with medical treatment.

RRT Method

Usually, when RRT is indicated, children with ALF are at risk of or have a multiorgan dysfunction syndrome, with hemodynamic, respiratory, renal, and neurological (intracranial hypertension with cerebral edema) failures and inflammation status (see chapters on Acute Liver Failure and Acute-on-Chronic Liver Failure). RRT is used to prevent/support those complications, to remove ammonia and to potentially decrease proinflammatory cytokines (e.g. tumor necrosis factor, interleukin also found in sepsis) [2, 11].

Continuous Renal Replacement Therapies

Continuous renal replacement therapies (CRRT) include continuous venovenous hemofiltration (CVVH), continuous venovenous hemodialysis (CVVHD), and continuous venovenous hemodiafiltration (CVVHDF). With all these modalities, small molecular weight toxins are removed, water removal (ultrafiltration) can be spread over 24 h resulting in a better hemodynamic tolerance, and osmolar shifts, at risk of cerebral herniation [10, 12], can be better controlled. High-volume hemofiltration (HVCVVH) i.e. $\geq$80 ml/kg/h is the preferred method in ALF as the convection modality can remove higher molecular weight molecules that can include cytokines, but it can be combined with dialysis (CVVHD) to increase small molecular weight toxin removal (ammonia for example) [13]. Using HVCVVH, Chevret et al. [14] reported an improvement in ammonia and bilirubin levels, decrease in serum creatinine, and improvement in encephalopathy grade.

Intermittent Hemodialysis

iHD can decrease ammonia level by 75% within 3–4 h faster than CRRT. Due to its intermittent nature, there is a risk of rebound and, in a condition such as ALF with constant toxins generation, iHD sessions are prolonged and usually repeated daily. Children on iHD are more at risk of hypotension episodes and osmolar shift that can worsen cerebral edema and increase the risk of cerebral herniation in ALF patient with intracranial hypertension [10, 15].

Peritoneal Dialysis

In the last century, this modality was the treatment of choice in children when iHD and CRRT were considered too dangerous for the neonates and children. However, advances in technology and techniques have now made iHD and CRRT safer and readily available in most pediatric centers. Due to its limited efficacy for toxins clearance and the increase of abdominal pressure due to dialysate volume, its use should be reserved when no other RRT are available [10, 15].

> High-volume continuous venovenous hemofiltration is the preferred renal replacement therapy in critically ill children with acute or acute-on-chronic liver failure.

Extracorporeal Liver Support Therapies

The extracorporeal liver support therapies are meant to mitigate the impact of liver failure and decrease mortality while hepatic cells regenerate [3, 6, 7]. This *bridge to recovery* can be associated with a better long-term survival [6, 16]. ELST can be initiated in severe ALF and ACLF with hepatic encephalopathy, hemodynamic instability, severe coagulopathy, renal dysfunction, infection, fluid overload, or severe pruritus [3, 5, 8]. The ESLT are divided in two categories: artificial liver support and bioartificial liver support.

Artificial Extracorporeal Liver Support Systems (Table 1)

Albumin Dialysis

Albumin dialysis is one of the main method studied for the management of ALF and ACLF. The rational of albumin dialysis is based on the restoration of the native albumin function by removing highly protein-bound toxins. Several methods currently exist using a combination of filtration and adsorption, and two menial devices are commercially available: MARS® and Prometheus® [3].

With the Molecular Adsorbents Recirculating System, MARS®, (Baxter, Stockholm, Sweden, 1996), the patient's blood passes through a first circuit comprising a hemofilter with a specialized semipermeable membrane, selective for <50–60 kDa molecules. In a second circuit operating in parallel, 20% albumin dialysate passes in a countercurrent, which promotes the passage of albumin-bound toxins from the patient's blood through the membrane to free sites on the unbound albumin. In turn, this toxin-filled dialysate is passed through a second semipermeable filter on a continuous renal replacement therapy (CRRT) device where the water-soluble toxins are removed by standard diffusion and convection. Albumin-bound toxins are then removed when the albumin passes through two adsorbent cartridges, activated charcoal and an anion resin, regenerating it before returning in the first hemofilter (Fig. 1). Two filters are available for MARS® depending on the patient's weight: one for patients weighing more than 25 kg (adult filter, 2.1 m^2, fill volume 152 mL) and one, the MARSmini, for children weighing less than 25 kg (0.6 m^2, fill volume 57 mL) [3, 16, 17].

Prometheus®, the Fractionated Plasma Separation and Adsorption system (FPSA) (Fresenius Medical Care, Bad Homburg, Germany, 1999), also consists of two circuits. The patient's blood first passes through an albumin-permeable membrane (with a cut-off of 250–300 kDa) where the patient's plasma is separated and similarly passes through two adsorption columns to remove albumin-bound toxins before returning in the blood compartment. The blood then passes through a regular dialysis machine for the removal of water-soluble toxins. This system is only intended for adult patients because of its large extracorporeal volume (700–750 ml)

Table 1 Comparison of seven extracorporeal methods used in children to remove toxins accumulated in acute liver failure

	CRRT	HV-CRRT	MARS®	Prometheus®	TPE/RRT	SPAD	ELAD/HepatAssist
Exchange mechanism(s)	Convection	Convection	Diffusion Adsorption	Plasma separation Adsorption Diffusion	Diffusion	Diffusion	Plasma separation Adsorption Diffusion
Molecular cut off (kDa)	~50	~50	~50	~900	~900	~50	~50–150
Advantages	Low complexity	Low complexity	Removal of protein-bound substance	Removal of protein-bound substance	Removal of protein-bound substance	Low complexity Removal of protein-bound substance	Removal of protein-bound substance
Benefits	Improve biochemical parameters	Reduce HE Improve biochemical parameters	Reduce HE Improve biochemical parameters	Reduce HE Improve biochemical parameters	Improve coagulopathy Improve biochemical parameters Survival improvement	Improve biochemical parameters	Improve neurological function
Disadvantages			Complexity	Complexity	Complexity	Albumin use	Complexity Use of hepatoblastoma cells Use of porcine hepatocytes
Pediatric RCT	0	0	0	0	0	0	0

Adapted from: Merouani and Jouvet [29]

CRRT Continuous Renal Replacement Therapy, *HV-CRRT* High-Volume – Continuous Renal Replacement Therapy, *MARS*® molecular absorbant recirculating system (Baxter, Stockholm, Sweden, 1996), *Prometheus*® Prometheus® dialysis (Fresenius Medical Care, Bad Homburg, Germany, 1999), *TPE/RRT* Therapeutic Plasma exchange: plasmapheresis combined with renal replacement therapy, *SPAD* Single-Pass Albumin Dialysis, *ELAD/HepatAssis* Extracorporeal liver assist device, human hepatocyte bioreactor (Vital Therapy, San Diego, California, USA)/HepatAssist: Porcine Hepatocyte bioreactor (Arbios, formerly Circe, Waltham, MA)

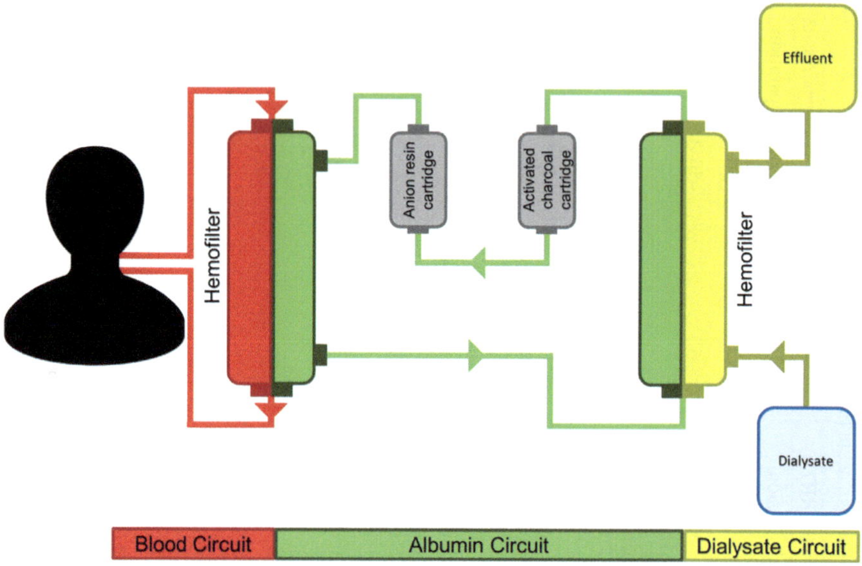

Fig. 1 Diagram of the molecular adsorbents recirculating system (MARS®)

[3, 18]. However, some authors have suggested a protocol for its pediatric use, based on local experience [19].

Single-Pass Albumin Dialysis (SPAD) is a method that uses a standard renal replacement system, usually CRRT, in which albumin is added to the dialysate to provide a 20% solution to improve the removal of albumin-bound toxins from the patient's blood, which would normally be limited. However, unlike MARS®, albumin is not recycled in this method and is wasted in the effluent. Therefore, this technique is primarily an alternative for newborns and infants since the total amount of dialysate used in a single treatment is lower and will represent a more reasonable amount of albumin to use.

Therapeutic Plasma Exchange (Plasmapheresis)

Various antibodies, circulating factors, and toxins can be removed by replacing the patient's plasma, including albumin-bound and unbound toxins (e.g. aromatic amino acids, ammonia, endotoxins, and others) from the intravascular compartment. Those treatments aim not only at toxins removal but also at coagulation factors correction and are hypothesized to replace dysfunctional and potentially inflammatory circulating abnormal albumin which can occur in more chronic conditions [20].

Two categories of devices are used for therapeutic plasma exchanges (TPE), either filtration through plasma separator (high cut-off hemofilter allowing for ultrafiltration of whole plasma), with cartridges useable on standard renal replacement therapy (RRT) machines, or by collection during centrifugation, requiring more specialized devices which also allow for different types of apheresis therapies. The majority of the patient's plasma is removed during each treatment and replaced, most commonly, with fresh frozen plasma (FFP) or albumin. This approach, when using FFP, also improves coagulopathy by correcting coagulation factors levels without increasing fluid overload.

Both standard (1 to 1.5x patient's plasma volume) and high volume exchanges (>2 patient's plasma volume) have been studied as supportive therapy for ALF [3, 21, 22]. While its use in ALF is often combined with RRT to improve toxins clearance, TPE has the advantage of being more readily available in large centers, as opposed to albumin dialysis which requires dedicated devices with a specific expertise.

Artificial Extracorporeal Liver Support Efficacy

Different parameters have been studied to evaluate the efficacy of the artificial extracorporeal liver support methods in ALF. However, only few sources have investigated pediatric cases, with small underpowered studies. Prometheus has not been studied in children, due to challenges with the large extracorporeal volume needed. Consistent with adult literature, pediatric studies showed improved biochemistry with MARS®, including decrease in serum bilirubin, bile acids, ammonia, urea, and creatinine [3]. However, these methods were not associated with clinical relevant outcomes improvement in adults.

The severity of hepatic encephalopathy and a significant reduction in intracranial pressure was also reported with the use of MARS®. Few studies comparing MARS® or Prometheus® to standard medical treatment have shown some improvement in the neurologic status of ALF patients. This effect was probably limited by the difficulties in neurological assessment of these patients, especially those undergoing mechanical ventilation and sedation [3, 23]. Difficulty in documenting the impact of artificial extracorporeal liver support methods on clinical outcome was also due to the short time period spent on the waiting list before LT [2, 6].

There are no large controlled trials to routinely recommend these methods to children with ALF, particularly in countries where liver transplantation is rapidly performed [3, 18, 24]. Although the pediatric literature is scarce, a recent meta-analysis of studies in adults reported a reduction in mortality with the use of ELSTs, all techniques combined, as well as an improvement in hepatic encephalopathy, with moderate and low certainty respectively [6]. However, potential bias may have mitigated the results, as the studies analyzed were often industry-funded, and all techniques were grouped together for analysis. Nevertheless, further studies are needed before formal recommendations can be made regarding artificial ELSTs.

Several studies have suggested a beneficial effect of TPE in improving neurological and biochemical parameters with an additional benefit on coagulopathy compared to albumin dialysis [17, 22]. High-volume TPE applied in patient with ALF has also been studied. Three exchanges of 15% of ideal body weight (8–12 L) over 3 days showed an improvement in survival compared to standard medical treatment in adults that did not, or could not have LT [22]. Plasma exchange alone may not improve clinical outcomes and survival in children, primarily because of the low volume of unbound toxins eliminated when treating the intravascular compartment alone with TPE, but encouraging evidence is present when combined with RRT in adults and in pediatric studies [3, 17, 22, 25]. However, comparable high-volume TPE have not been studied in children. European recommendations for adults specify that the use of plasma exchange may be of greater benefit if patients are treated early and will not have LT at term [2, 6, 23].

> Among artificial extracorporeal liver support systems, therapeutic plasma exchange might improve the outcome of critically ill children with severe acute or acute-on-chronic liver failure, in combination with high-volume continuous venovenous hemofiltration.

Biological Extracorporeal Liver Support Systems

Theses supports combine two techniques: plasma separation and perfusion of biocells containing either engineered human hepatoblastoma cells or freshly isolated porcine hepatocytes. Bioreactors used consist in a column containing hollow capillary fibers with semipermeable membrane (cut-off of 50-150 kDa) allowing for patient's plasma to come in contact with hepatocytes in the extracapillary space. Those hepatic cells can survive 3 to 10 days during the treatment and mimic in vivo function like albumin synthesis and cytochrome P450 activity. Some devices also warm and oxygenate the patient's blood [26]. Cells' viability and their metabolism are very important for the metabolites exchange. In addition to the detoxification, one of the main advantages of biological supports is the replication of metabolic and biosynthetic functions of hepatic cells [3, 5, 25, 27]. Three devices are used in experimental trials and no pediatric clinical trial has been done:

- SRBAL, spheroid reservoir bio-artificial liver [27]
- ELAD, extracorporeal liver assist device, (Vital Therapy, San Diego, California, USA): human hepatocyte bioreactor
- HepatAssist (Arbios, formerly Circe, Waltham, MA), Porcine Hepatocyte bioreactor.

Only few small and uncontrolled studies have been conducted in humans with biological extracorporeal liver support systems. They showed an improvement in neurological function and provided a bridge to LT, but there was no evidence of significant improvement in mean blood pressure, ammonia and bilirubin levels, encephalopathy or renal function, and no improvement in survival [28]. These studies have been conducted on adults, none in children to date [3, 26], and further research is needed.

Conclusion

Acute liver failure is a complex disease that requires the investigation and management of its underlying etiology, as well as the prevention and support of its complications. To support the liver until its recovery or LT, multiple extracorporeal liver devices have been studied. Most of the current data are from adult patients, often with acute-on-chronic failure, and are therefore not applicable to most children. The management of children with ALF remains primarily focused on supporting the various organs failures (e.g. kidneys, lungs and brain). No recent guidelines have recommended the systematic use of ELST in ALF patients. These devices are generally not readily available outside of study protocols or from certain highly specialized centers. Plasma exchange therapies are the only technique that has been promoted by the European Association for the Study of the Liver with survival benefit. In addition, ALF is a rare disease in pediatric intensive care units, and the critical mass of patients required to maintain clinical expertise on these specialized devices may not be sufficient. The lack of strong recommendations, and often clinical expertise, for specialized therapies such as albumin dialysis often directs clinical teams to forms of ELST that use more familiar and readily methods i.e. CRRT and TPE.

Bioartificial systems represent an interesting area and their potential benefits on patient metabolic states could be of great help in the management of children with ALF in pediatric intensive care units. However, those devices are still being studied and require further investigation.

References

1. Tissieres P, Devictor D. Acute liver failure and liver transplantation. In: Rogers' textbook of pediatric intensive care. 5th ed. Wolters Kluwer; 2008.
2. EASL. Clinical practical guidelines on the management of acute (fulminant) liver failure. J Hepatol. 2017;66(5):1047–81.
3. Jain V, Dhawan A. Extracorporeal liver support systems in paediatric liver failure. J Pediatr Gastroenterol Nutr. 2017;64(6):855–63.
4. Warrillow S, Bellomo R. Intensive care management of severe acute liver failure. Annu Update Intensive Care Emerg Med. 2015;2015(2015):415–30.
5. Katarey D, Jalan R. Update on extracorporeal liver support. Curr Opin Crit Care. 2020;26(2):180–5.
6. Alshamsi F, Alshammari K, Belley-Cote E, Dionne J, Albrahim T, Albudoor B, et al. Extracorporeal liver support in patients with liver failure: a systematic review and meta-analysis of randomized trials. Intensive Care Med. 2020;46(1):1–16.
7. Wiesmann T, Hoenl D, Wulf H, Irqsusi M. Extracorporeal liver support: trending epidemiology and mortality - a nationwide database analysis 2007-2015. BMC Gastroenterol. 2019;19(1):160.
8. Singanayagam A, Bernal W. Update on acute liver failure. Curr Opin Crit Care. 2015;21(2):134–41.
9. Alfadhel M, Mutairi FA, Makhseed N, Jasmi FA, Al-Thihli K, Al-Jishi E, et al. Guidelines for acute management of hyperammonemia in the Middle East region. Ther Clin Risk Manag. 2016;12:479–87.

10. Raina R, Bedoyan JK, Lichter-Konecki U, Jouvet P, Picca S, Mew NA, et al. Consensus guidelines for management of hyperammonaemia in paediatric patients receiving continuous kidney replacement therapy. Nat Rev Nephrol. 2020;16(8):471–82.
11. Slack AJ, Auzinger G, Willars C, Dew T, Musto R, Corsilli D, et al. Ammonia clearance with haemofiltration in adults with liver disease. Liver Int. 2014;34(1):42–8.
12. Liotta EM, Romanova AL, Lizza BD, Rasmussen-Torvik LJ, Kim M, Francis B, et al. Osmotic shifts, cerebral edema, and neurologic deterioration in severe hepatic encephalopathy. Crit Care Med. 2018;46(2):280–9.
13. Spinale JM, Laskin BL, Sondheimer N, Swartz SJ, Goldstein SL. High-dose continuous renal replacement therapy for neonatal hyperammonemia. Pediatr Nephrol. 2013;28(6):983–6.
14. Chevret L, Durand P, Lambert J, Essouri S, Balu L, Devictor D, et al. High-volume hemofiltration in children with acute liver failure. Pediatr Crit Care Med. 2014;15(7):e300.
15. Gupta S, Fenves AZ, Hootkins R. The role of RRT in hyperammonemic patients. Clin J Am Soc Nephrol CJASN. 2016;11(10):1872–8.
16. Saliba F, Camus C, Durand F, Mathurin P, Letierce A, Delafosse B, et al. Albumin dialysis with a noncell artificial liver support device in patients with acute liver failure. Ann Intern Med. 2013;159(8):522–31.
17. Ide K, Muguruma T, Shinohara M, Toida C, Enomoto Y, Matsumoto S, et al. Continuous venovenous hemodiafiltration and plasma exchange in infantile acute liver failure. Pediatr Crit Care Med. 2015;16(8):e268.
18. Novelli G, Rossi M, Morabito V, Pugliese F, Ruberto F, Perrella SM, et al. Pediatric acute liver failure with molecular adsorbent recirculating system treatment. Transplant Proc. 2008;40(6):1921–4.
19. Walle JV, Claus S, Snauwaert E, Rudder JD, Raes A, Dick M, et al. Prometheus® liver therapy in children with acute liver failure. Crit Care. 2015;19(Suppl 1):P381.
20. Jalan R, Schnurr K, Mookerjee RP, Sen S, Cheshire L, Hodges S, et al. Alterations in the functional capacity of albumin in patients with decompensated cirrhosis is associated with increased mortality. Hepatology. 2009;50(2):555–64.
21. Akcan Arikan A, Srivaths P, Himes RW, Tufan Pekkucuksen N, Lam F, Nguyen T, et al. Hybrid extracorporeal therapies as a bridge to pediatric liver transplantation. Pediatr Crit Care Med. 2018;19(7):e342–9.
22. Larsen FS, Schmidt LE, Bernsmeier C, Rasmussen A, Isoniemi H, Patel VC, et al. High-volume plasma exchange in patients with acute liver failure: an open randomised controlled trial. J Hepatol. 2016;64(1):69–78.
23. Fuhrmann V, Bauer M, Wilmer A. The persistent potential of extracorporeal therapies in liver failure. Intensive Care Med. 2020;46(3):528–30.
24. Covic A, Goldsmith DJA, Gusbeth-Tatomir P, Volovat C, Dimitriu AG, Cristogel F, et al. Successful use of molecular absorbent regenerating system (MARS) dialysis for the treatment of fulminant hepatic failure in children accidentally poisoned by toxic mushroom ingestion. Liver Int. 2003;23(s3):21–7.
25. Schaefer B, Schaefer F, Engelmann G, Meyburg J, Heckert KH, Zorn M, et al. Comparison of molecular adsorbents recirculating system (MARS) dialysis with combined plasma exchange and haemodialysis in children with acute liver failure. Nephrol Dial Transplant. 2011;26(11):3633–9.
26. Jalan R, Sen S, Williams R. Prospects for extracorporeal liver support. Gut. 2004;53(6):890–8.
27. Chen HS, Joo DJ, Shaheen M, Li Y, Wang Y, Yang J, et al. Randomized trial of spheroid reservoir bioartificial liver in porcine model of posthepatectomy liver failure. Hepatology. 2019;69(1):329–42.
28. He Y-T, Qi Y-N, Zhang B-Q, Li J-B, Bao J. Bioartificial liver support systems for acute liver failure: a systematic review and meta-analysis of the clinical and preclinical literature. World J Gastroenterol. 2019;25(27):3634–48.
29. Merouani A, Jouvet P. High-volume hemofiltration for critically ill children with acute liver failure: a standard treatment? with permission. Pediatr Crit Care Med. 2014;15(7):681–3.

Liver Failure and the Lungs

Atsushi Kawaguchi and Philippe Jouvet

Introduction

Children with acute or acute-on-chronic liver failure (LF) may have an acute respiratory failure (ARF) following one or several simultaneous insults including hepatic encephalopathy, volume overload, pulmonary hemorrhage, pulmonary edema, acute lung injury (sepsis for instance), and other comorbidities such as ascites with intra-abdominal hypertension, hydrothorax, and muscle weakness due to poor nutritional conditions. The incidence of respiratory failure in critically ill children with LF varies among the reports from 20% to 50% [1–3]. Although it is not incorporated in the PELD score, respiratory failure and the needs for mechanical ventilation are associated with a higher mortality rate [4–6].

In the following sections, we focus on five pathophysiological conditions associated with liver diseases (i.e., lung inflammation, intra-abdominal hypertension (IAH), hepatopulmonary syndrome (HPS), porto-pulmonary hypertension (POPH), and hepatic hydrothorax).

A. Kawaguchi (✉)
Department of Pediatrics, CHU Sainte-Justine, University of Montreal, Montreal, QC, Canada

Department of Intensive Care Medicine, Tokyo Women's Medical University, Tokyo, Japan

P. Jouvet
Pediatric Intensive Care Unit - Department of Pediatrics of Sainte Justine Hospital, University of Montreal, Montréal, QC, Canada

P. Jouvet, F. Alvarez (eds.), *Liver Diseases in the Pediatric Intensive Care Unit*, https://doi.org/10.1007/978-3-030-79132-2_7

Lung Inflammation

In children with LF, lung inflammation is mainly due to a sepsis (pneumonia, peritonitis, catheter-related bloodstream infection) and/or a systemic inflammatory response syndrome (SIRS) that results in lung edema and a hypoxic respiratory failure. The clinical diagnosis of lung inflammation corresponds to the pediatric acute respiratory distress syndrome (PARDS) definition as reported by the Pediatric Acute Lung Injury Consensus Conference [7] and is the most frequent ARF etiology in children with LF.

PARDS Management

In the absence of specific recommendations for the management of PARDS in LF, the ventilatory support should include a lung-protective strategy with low tidal volume, and restricted plateau pressure [7]. Besides, careful attention should be procured to the permissive hypercapnia level in the management of children with LF who frequently have an increased intracranial pressure due to cerebral edema. In such a situation, the monitoring of intracranial perfusion using intracranial Doppler could be helpful. Ventilatory management with sufficient positive end-expiratory pressure (PEEP) should be central to avoid lung collapse at higher closing pressures during expiration. However, the appropriate PEEP level setting needs also to take into account the possibility of a high cardiac output failure, intra-abdominal hypertension, or pulmonary hypertension. In the context of malnutrition and systemic muscle weakness including diaphragmatic fatigue, we could also consider the novel techniques in respiratory management to enhance diaphragm muscle activity such as esophageal transpulmonary pressure catheter and electric activity of the diaphragm [8].

> Several associated conditions need to be taken into consideration for the management of PARDS in children with liver failure including intracranial hypertension, high cardiac output failure, pulmonary hypertension.

Intra-abdominal Hypertension

Excessive ascites and enlarged liver are frequent complications in children with LF, which could contribute to IAH. IAH causes an elevation of the diaphragm affecting lung volumes and respiratory mechanics (Table 1) [9–14]. The effects of IAH on respiratory function can be mainly characterized by a decrease in respiratory system compliance and an increase of intrathoracic pressure affecting airway, pleural, and central vascular pressures. Here, abdominal-thoracic transmission (ATT) describes

Table 1 Effects of intra-abdominal hypertension on respiratory mechanics

Intra-thoracic pressure ↑	
Pleural pressure	↑
Peak airway pressure with volume controlled MV	↑
Mean airway pressure	↑
Plateau airway pressure	↑
Compression atelectasis	↑
Pulmonary vascular resistance	↑
Lower inflection points on pressure volume curve	↑
Respiratory system compliance ↓ due to chest wall compliance ↓	
Functional residual capacity (FRC)	↓
Lung volume in pressure controlled mode	↓

the proportion of an increase in thoracic pressures for each incremental elevation of intra-abdominal pressure. ATT of peak and plateau airway pressure has been reported to be between 20% and 60% [14, 15]. This ATT can lead to increased work of breathing with reduced functional residual capacity and lower lung volumes. IAH by itself may cause lung edema resulting in poor oxygenation and ventilation with increased dead space and ventilation-perfusion mismatch. IAH may also result in ventilator-induced acute lung injury with increased shear stress with or without systemic inflammatory response or chemical aspiration.

Diagnosis and Management of IAH

The gold standard for intra-abdominal pressure (IAP) measurement is through a peritoneal catheter, which is invasive and technically challenging in children. IAP can be indirectly measured using a bladder method, which is closely correlated with IAP [16]. The bladder pressure should be taken at end-expiration after allowing time for equilibration of bladder pressures and ensuring the absence of abdominal muscle contractions. Normal IAP in children on positive pressure ventilation is below 8 mmHg. IAH is defined as a sustained IAP greater than 10 mmHg [9].

The goal of IAH management in critically ill children is to prevent further organ dysfunction including respiratory failure and prevention of abdominal compartment syndrome. Ventilatory support is based on lung protective strategies as recommended by the Pediatric Acute Lung Injury Consensus Conference [7]. In some cases, it may be necessary to use muscle relaxants to improve thoracic compliance.

> The intra-abdominal pressure can be indirectly measured using a bladder catheter.

Hepatopulmonary Syndrome

HPS is recognized as a pulmonary vascular disorder associated with portal hypertension or congenital porto-systemic shunts. Pathophysiology of HPS is characterized by an increased alveolar-arterial (A-a) gradient with a significant dilation of the pulmonary artery and capillary vessels. Clinically, HPS is defined by the triad of an increase of A-a gradient, the presence of liver disease, and evidence for intrapulmonary vascular dilation which can be observed by echocardiography. In particular, significant pulmonary vascular dilation increases the venous blood flow leading to ventilation–perfusion mismatch relative to unchanged alveolar ventilation (Fig. 1). Another observed feature of HPS is a platypnea-orthodeoxia syndrome which is a positional dyspnea and hypoxemia stemmed from intracardiac shunting, pulmonary shunting, ventilation-perfusion mismatch, or a combination of these. This seems to be due to the overproduction of nitric oxide (NO), endothelin-1 (ET-1), intestinal endotoxemia increasing tumor necrosis factor, heme-oxygenase-1, and endothelial-derived hyperpolarizing factor [17–21].

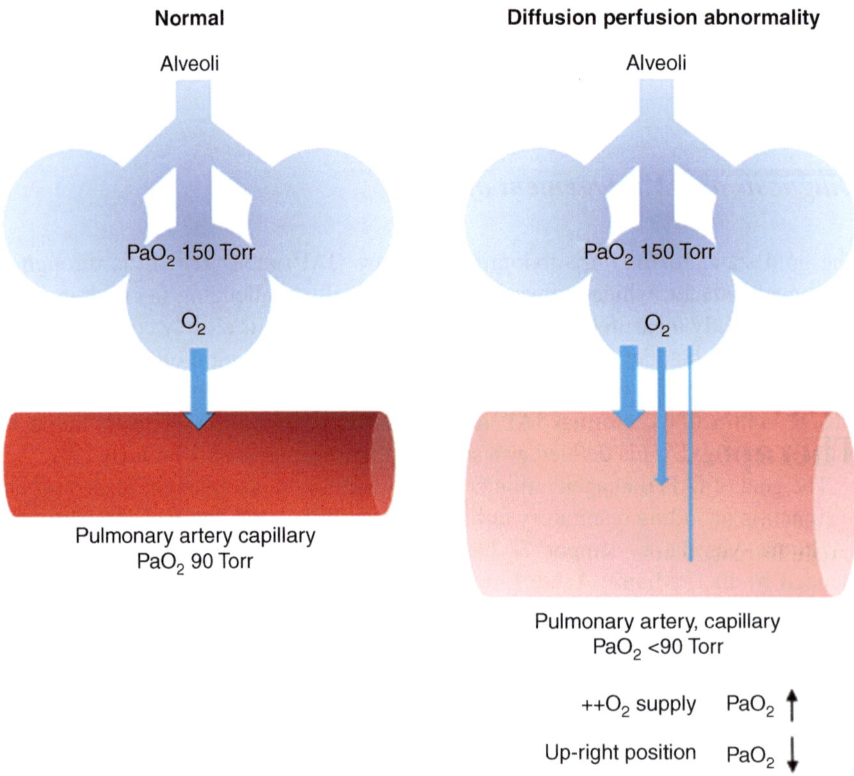

Fig. 1 Pathophysiology of hypoxemia in hepatopulmonary syndrome

Diagnosis and Management of HPS

HPS can be diagnosed with the following three criteria: (1) the presence of liver disease and/or portal hypertension; (2) elevated room air alveolar-arterial oxygen gradient (≥15 mmHg); and (3) evidence of intrapulmonary vascular dilations [22], which should be based on arterial blood gas analyses and A-a gradient calculation (Table 2). The contrast-enhanced echocardiography with agitated saline is considered the gold standard for the evaluation of intrapulmonary vasodilation, and the use of macro-aggregates of albumin allows to quantify the pulmonary shunts.

Liver transplantation is the only treatment potentially able to modify the HPS, meaning medical management of HPS is basically considered as supportive management. Several pharmaceutical interventions have been examined without encouraging outcomes, in which NO-mediated pulmonary vasodilation and angiogenesis induced by proinflammatory cytokines have been the main targets of the intervention. Although those have not been well examined in children, the drugs tested included such as octreotide (a somatostatin analogue inhibiting angiogenesis), pentoxifylline (TNF-α inhibitor), and sorafenib (reducing VEGF-mediated angiogenesis and down-regulating eNOS activation through tyrosine kinase receptor inhibition) [23–26]. Although those have not been well examined in children. Other interventions as treatment with the norfloxacin [27, 28], methylene blue [29, 30], almitrine bismesylate and garlic supplementation that inhibit NO synthesis [31, 32] have not shown promising results in clinical trials even in the adult cohorts.

Invasive interventions such as portal decompression with trans-jugular intrahepatic portosystemic shunting have been tested with mitigated results [33, 34]. Embolotherapy has also been examined in the presence of major arteriovenous communications [35, 36].

The evidence of severe hypoxemia in HPS (PaO_2 <60 mm Hg) should be considered an indication for orthotopic liver transplantation (OLT) [37].

> Hepatopulmonary syndrome diagnosis is based on an elevated room air alveolar-arterial oxygen gradient (≥15 mmHg).

Table 2 Diagnosis criteria of hepatopulmonary syndrome

1	Liver disease and/or portal hypertension
2	Alveolar-arterial oxygen gradient ≥15 mmHg on room air OR partial pressure oxygen (PaO_2) <80 mmHg on room air Staging of HPS 1. Mild PaO_2 ≥80 mmHg 2. Moderate PaO_2 60–79 mmHg 3. Severe PaO_2 50–59 mmHg 4. Very severe PaO_2 <50 mmHg
3	Presence of pulmonary vascular dilation documented by (1) contrast-enhanced transthoracic echocardiography OR (2) lung perfusion scanning with radioactive albumin

All the three criteria need to be met

Porto-Pulmonary Hypertension

POPH is defined by the presence of a mean pulmonary artery pressure above 25 mmHg at rest and a pulmonary capillary wedge pressure less than 15 mmHg in adult cohorts [17–20]. The incidence of POPH is ranging from 0.5% to 6% in patients with portal hypertension or congenital porto-systemic shunts, but there is no sufficient data in pediatric cases. Studies suggest that the prognosis of untreated POPH is dismal compared with the patients without POPH, although most of the available data stem from either small adult retrospective observational study.

Several underlining pathophysiology have been reported including an imbalance of vascular mediators associated with vasoconstriction, endothelial damage with vascular remodeling due to excessive pulmonary blood flow, smooth muscle proliferation, and microvascular thrombosis [17]. Hypoxemia and a decreased carbon dioxide level could be observed in arterial blood gases, which is less pronounced than in HPS.

Diagnosis and Management of POPH

Children with POPH are often asymptomatic. Therefore, an echocardiography screening for POPH should be performed in all children being evaluated for LT or patients with portal hypertension or congenital porto-systemic shunts, even without signs or symptoms [38]. Cardiac catheterization should be considered in children with signs of pulmonary arterial hypertension (PAH) for the definitive diagnosis of POPH. Children with severe liver disease should have other reasons than liver failure itself for an increase of pulmonary pressure, such as volume overload, primary lung disease, chronic hypoxia, chronic thromboembolic PAH, and hyperdynamic cardiac state (see Liver and Heart chapter). When volume overload and/or hyperdynamic cardiac state are present, pulmonary arterial wedge pressure and/or cardiac index should be often evaluated. Transpulmonary pressure gradient which can be calculated with mean pulmonary arterial pressure (PAP) and pulmonary arterial occlusion pressure, >12 mmHg are in favor of POPH rather than PAH with hyperdynamic cardiac state [22, 39]. Findings of hypoxemia in blood gas analysis and elevation of plasma biomarkers such as B-type natriuretic peptide may also help the diagnosis but are not specific.

Treatments and Transplant Consideration

Same as in cases with HPS, supplementary MELD points could be assigned to LT candidates with POPH, particularly when responding to the following selective pulmonary vasodilator therapy. It should also be noted that LT itself in the setting of POPH remains at higher risk, and the resolution of POPH post-transplant is unpredictable. In other words, LT could precipitate acute cardiac failure, the probability of which is much higher in those with an already compromised right ventricle function. Some adult studies suggested that a PAP >50 mmHg should be considered as a contraindication for LT [39, 40].

There is no standardized approach for POPH. The PAH therapies have been applied to patients with POPH taking into account the possible presence of liver parenchymal disease. For instance, anticoagulation and calcium channel blockers, which have been widely recommended in PAH patients, should be a contraindication for those with POPH due to abnormal coagulation and potential mesenteric dilation properties which may result in worsening of portal hypertension.

The oxygen therapy and fluid management should follow the same rules as for PAH. Currently, three different pathways have been targeted in PAH medical therapies: (1) proteinoids (potent pulmonary and systemic vasodilators as well as inhibitors of platelet aggregation), (2) endothelin receptor antagonists (potent vasoconstrictor molecule), and (3) phosphodiesterase type 5 inhibitors. However, the benefits of those new therapies in POPH cases, particularly in children, are still unknown due to the lack of high-quality interventional controlled trials [41].

> Children with porto-pulmonary hypertension are often asymptomatic and need an echocardiography screening in all children being evaluated for LT.

Hepatic Hydrothorax

As a result of portal hypertension or mal-nutrition, excessive ascites can be commonly observed in children with LF. HH is defined by the presence of ascites in the pleural cavity without evidence of other disease etiology causing pleural effusion [5, 18–20]. HH results from the transitioning of excessive ascites via a small defect in the diaphragm which more commonly occurs in the right side of the chest cavity. It is also reported that HH can be observed without ascites that was explained by the negative intrathoracic pressure on inspiration. For children with HH, the main treatment strategy can be salt restriction and diuretics similar to known medical treatment of ascites. Repeated thoracentesis and trans-jugular intrahepatic portosystemic shunt can be considered as an option in children too. Some reports suggested repair of the diaphragmatic defects as an option in case of no indication or contraindication for a liver transplantation; however, such a repair could be technically challenging in children [5, 18–20, 42].

Conclusions

When children with liver disease suffer from respiratory distress or failure, it is important to carefully evaluate all the possible causes as they can be intertwined. Although the basic concepts of respiratory management are similar for all conditions (e.g., lung protective strategies in PARDS, decreased abdominal pressure in IAH), they need to be adapted to other clinical conditions observed in LF (e.g., intracranial hypertension, high cardiac output failure). Further researches are needed to better manage this specific association of lung damage and liver failure.

References

1. Bhatt H, Rao GS. Management of acute liver failure: a pediatric perspective. Curr Pediatr Rep. 2018;6(3):246–57.
2. Lutfi R, Abulebda K, Nitu ME, Molleston JP, Bozic MA, Subbarao G. Intensive care management of pediatric acute liver failure. J Pediatr Gastroenterol Nutr. 2017;64(5):660–70.
3. Squires JE, McKiernan P, Squires RH. Acute liver failure: an update. Clin Liver Dis. 2018;22(4):773–805.
4. Boente RD, Sheikh A, Bosslet GT, Ghabril MS. Outcomes of acute respiratory distress syndrome in mechanically ventilated patients with cirrhosis. Crit Care Explor. 2019;1(9):e0040.
5. Devictor D, Tissieres P, Afanetti M, Debray D. Acute liver failure in children. Clin Res Hepatol Gastroenterol. 2011;35(6–7):430–7.
6. Wiesner RH, McDiarmid SV, Kamath PS, Edwards EB, Malinchoc M, Kremers WK, et al. MELD and PELD: application of survival models to liver allocation. Liver Transpl. 2001;7(7):567–80.
7. Pediatric Acute Lung Injury Consensus Conference Group. Pediatric acute respiratory distress syndrome: consensus recommendations from the pediatric acute lung injury consensus conference. Pediatr Crit Care Med. 2015;16(5):428–39.
8. Rafferty GF, Greenough A, Manczur T, Polkey MI, Harris ML, Heaton ND, et al. Magnetic phrenic nerve stimulation to assess diaphragm function in children following liver transplantation. Pediatr Crit Care Med. 2001;2(2):122–6.
9. Thabet FC, Ejike JC. Intra-abdominal hypertension and abdominal compartment syndrome in pediatrics. A review. J Crit Care. 2017;41:275–82.
10. Bressan AK, Ball CG. Intra-abdominal hypertension and abdominal compartment syndrome in acute pancreatitis, hepato-pancreato-biliary operations and liver transplantation. Anaesthesiol Intensive Ther. 2017;49(2):159–66.
11. Maluso P, Olson J, Sarani B. Abdominal compartment hypertension and abdominal compartment syndrome. Crit Care Clin. 2016;32(2):213–22.
12. Kirkpatrick AW, Roberts DJ, De Waele J, Jaeschke R, Malbrain ML, De Keulenaer B, et al. Intra-abdominal hypertension and the abdominal compartment syndrome: updated consensus definitions and clinical practice guidelines from the World Society of the Abdominal Compartment Syndrome. Intensive Care Med. 2013;39(7):1190–206.
13. Hedenstierna G, Larsson A. Influence of abdominal pressure on respiratory and abdominal organ function. Curr Opin Crit Care. 2012;18(1):80–5.
14. Regli A, Pelosi P, Malbrain M. Ventilation in patients with intra-abdominal hypertension: what every critical care physician needs to know. Ann Intensive Care. 2019;9(1):52.
15. Fiedler MO, Deutsch BL, Simeliunas E, Diktanaite D, Harms A, Brune M, et al. Effect of moderate elevated intra-abdominal pressure on lung mechanics and histological lung injury at different positive end-expiratory pressures. PLoS One. 2020;15(4):e0230830.
16. Davis PJ, Koottayi S, Taylor A, Butt WW. Comparison of indirect methods of measuring intra-abdominal pressure in children. Intensive Care Med. 2005;31(3):471–5.
17. Hoeper MM, Krowka MJ, Strassburg CP. Portopulmonary hypertension and hepatopulmonary syndrome. Lancet. 2004;363(9419):1461–8.
18. Qadir N, Wang T, Barjaktarevic I, Chang SY. Acute respiratory failure and pulmonary complications in end-stage liver disease. Semin Respir Crit Care Med. 2018;39(5):546–55.

19. Ramalingam VS, Ansari S, Fisher M. Respiratory complication in liver disease. Crit Care Clin. 2016;32(3):357–69.
20. Hemprich U, Papadakos PJ, Lachmann B. Respiratory failure and hypoxemia in the cirrhotic patient including hepatopulmonary syndrome. Curr Opin Anaesthesiol. 2010;23(2):133–8.
21. Cheng TO. Platypnea-orthodeoxia syndrome: etiology, differential diagnosis, and management. Catheter Cardiovasc Interv. 1999;47(1):64–6.
22. Rodriguez-Roisin R, Krowka MJ, Herve P, Fallon MB, Committee ERSTFP-HVDS. Pulmonary-hepatic vascular disorders (PHD). Eur Respir J. 2004;24(5):861–80.
23. Soderman C, Juhlin-Dannfelt A, Lagerstrand L, Eriksson LS. Ventilation-perfusion relationships and central haemodynamics in patients with cirrhosis. Effects of a somatostatin analogue. J Hepatol. 1994;21(1):52–7.
24. Yang W, Zhang J, Hu B, Wu W, Venter J, Alpini G, et al. The role of receptor tyrosine kinase activation in cholangiocytes and pulmonary vascular endothelium in experimental hepatopulmonary syndrome. Am J Physiol Gastrointest Liver Physiol. 2014;306(1):G72–80.
25. Chang CC, Chuang CL, Lee FY, Wang SS, Lin HC, Huang HC, et al. Sorafenib treatment improves hepatopulmonary syndrome in rats with biliary cirrhosis. Clin Sci (Lond). 2013;124(7):457–66.
26. Zhang J, Ling Y, Tang L, Luo B, Chacko BK, Patel RP, et al. Pentoxifylline attenuation of experimental hepatopulmonary syndrome. J Appl Physiol (1985). 2007;102(3):949–55.
27. Anel RM, Sheagren JN. Novel presentation and approach to management of hepatopulmonary syndrome with use of antimicrobial agents. Clin Infect Dis. 2001;32(10):E131–6.
28. Gupta S, Faughnan ME, Lilly L, Hutchison S, Fowler R, Bayoumi AM. Norfloxacin therapy for hepatopulmonary syndrome: a pilot randomized controlled trial. Clin Gastroenterol Hepatol. 2010;8(12):1095–8.
29. Miyamoto A, Katsuta Y, Zhang XJ, Li HL, Ohsuga M, Komeichi H, et al. Effect of chronic methylene blue administration on hypoxemia in rats with common bile duct ligation. Hepatol Res. 2010;40(6):622–32.
30. Rolla G, Bucca C, Brussino L. Methylene blue in the hepatopulmonary syndrome. N Engl J Med. 1994;331(16):1098.
31. Abrams GA, Fallon MB. Treatment of hepatopulmonary syndrome with Allium sativum L. (garlic): a pilot trial. J Clin Gastroenterol. 1998;27(3):232–5.
32. De BK, Dutta D, Pal SK, Gangopadhyay S, Das Baksi S, Pani A. The role of garlic in hepatopulmonary syndrome: a randomized controlled trial. Can J Gastroenterol. 2010;24(3):183–8.
33. Allgaier HP, Haag K, Ochs A, Hauenstein KH, Jeserich M, Krause T, et al. Hepato-pulmonary syndrome: successful treatment by transjugular intrahepatic portosystemic stent-shunt (TIPS). J Hepatol. 1995;23(1):102.
34. Paramesh AS, Husain SZ, Shneider B, Guller J, Tokat I, Gondolesi GE, et al. Improvement of hepatopulmonary syndrome after transjugular intrahepatic portasystemic shunting: case report and review of literature. Pediatr Transplant. 2003;7(2):157–62.
35. Poterucha JJ, Krowka MJ, Dickson ER, Cortese DA, Stanson AW, Krom RA. Failure of hepatopulmonary syndrome to resolve after liver transplantation and successful treatment with embolotherapy. Hepatology. 1995;21(1):96–100.
36. Lee HW, Suh KS, Kim J, Shin WY, Yi NJ, Jae HJ, et al. Pulmonary artery embolotherapy in a patient with type I hepatopulmonary syndrome after liver transplantation. Korean J Radiol. 2010;11(4):485–9.
37. Organ procurement and transplantation network. https://optn.transplant.hrsa.gov/media/1200/optn_policies.pdf. Accessed Jan 2021.
38. Galie N, Humbert M, Vachiery JL, Gibbs S, Lang I, Torbicki A, et al. 2015 ESC/ERS Guidelines for the diagnosis and treatment of pulmonary hypertension: The Joint Task Force for the Diagnosis and Treatment of Pulmonary Hypertension of the European Society of Cardiology (ESC) and the European Respiratory Society (ERS): Endorsed by: Association for European Paediatric and Congenital Cardiology (AEPC), International Society for Heart and Lung Transplantation (ISHLT). Eur Heart J. 2016;37(1):67–119.

39. Krowka MJ. Portopulmonary hypertension. Semin Respir Crit Care Med. 2012;33(1):17–25.
40. AbuHalimeh B, Krowka MJ, Tonelli AR. Treatment barriers in portopulmonary hypertension. Hepatology. 2019;69(1):431–43.
41. Hansmann G, Koestenberger M, Alastalo TP, Apitz C, Austin ED, Bonnet D, et al. 2019 updated consensus statement on the diagnosis and treatment of pediatric pulmonary hypertension: The European Pediatric Pulmonary Vascular Disease Network (EPPVDN), endorsed by AEPC, ESPR and ISHLT. J Heart Lung Transplant. 2019;38(9):879–901.
42. Karcz M, Bankey B, Schwaiberger D, Lachmann B, Papadakos PJ. Acute respiratory failure complicating advanced liver disease. Semin Respir Crit Care Med. 2012;33(1):96–110.

Liver Failure and the Heart

Sylvain Balandier, Karen Harrington, and Jean-Sébastien Joyal

Introduction

The liver is one of the most densely vascularized organs in the human body and is in immediate proximity to the heart. A veritable blood reservoir, it contains over 10% of the total blood volume in adults, and is traversed by 1.5 L of blood per minute, which represents 25% of total cardiac output. Any significant alteration in cardiac function may adversely impact the liver, and hepatic dysfunction has deleterious effects on the heart.

The Heart and the Liver: Anatomic Relationships

Blood flows to the liver via two major vessels, the hepatic artery and the portal vein. The hepatic artery carrying oxygenated blood from the aorta normally represents 20–30% of blood flow to the liver. The portal vein carries deoxygenated blood from the confluence of the superior mesenteric, inferior mesenteric, and splenic vein, and represents 70–80% of blood flow to the liver. A compensatory mechanism in the hepatic arterial circulation permits to increase its flow in response to decrease portal venous flow, and vice versa, which ensures stability of hepatic blood supply despite variations in portal flow. Venous outflow from the liver occurs via three hepatic veins draining the right, middle, and left parts of the liver, which join the inferior vena cava.

S. Balandier · K. Harrington (✉) · J.-S. Joyal
Pediatric Intensive Care Unit, Department of Pediatrics, CHU Sainte-Justine, Université de Montréal, Montreal, QC, Canada
e-mail: karen.harrington.med@ssss.gouv.qc.ca; jean-sebastien.joyal.med@ssss.gouv.qc.ca

P. Jouvet, F. Alvarez (eds.), *Liver Diseases in the Pediatric Intensive Care Unit*,
https://doi.org/10.1007/978-3-030-79132-2_8

Cardiac Complications of Pediatric Liver Diseases

High-Output Cardiac Failure

Kowalski and Abelmann [1] first described a hyperdynamic circulatory syndrome in patients with cirrhosis in 1953. Portal hypertension, decreased systemic vascular resistance, and increased cardiac output are the hallmarks of this gradual onset complication [2–4]. While understanding of the pathophysiology of cirrhotic hyperdynamic state remains incomplete, increased endogenous nitric oxide (NO) is recognized to have a major role [5].

Pathophysiology

Several interrelated mechanisms are involved: In the setting of portal hypertension, eNOS activity increases and increases circulating NO. NO-mediated splanchnic and peripheral arterial vasodilation cause effective central hypovolemia, while increased splanchnic flow maintains portal hypertension. Activation of the renin-angiotensin-aldosterone system mediates sodium and water retention, increasing circulating volume. Carotid baroceptors respond to central hypovolemia by increasing sympathetic nervous system activity, thus increasing cardiac inotropy and chronotropy [1–3].

While NO is central to the arterial vasodilation of cirrhotic hyperdynamic circulation, other circulating endogenous vasodilators contribute to, and may be increased by more production, impaired hepatic metabolism, and/or bypass of hepatic clearance via porto-systemic shunts. Prostacyclin, carbon monoxide, endogenous cannabinoids, endotoxin, and TNF alpha have all been the subject of study [4–6].

Clinical Presentation

Hyperdynamic circulation presents with tachycardia, systemic vasodilation, bounding pulses and widened systolic-diastolic pulse gradient. Cardiac output measurements show increased cardiac output and decreased systemic vascular resistance.

Cirrhotic patients are highly susceptible to hyperdynamic hemodynamic decompensation, mainly in the event of acute on chronic liver failure.

Treatment

Hyperdynamic circulation associated with cirrhosis is ultimately treated by correcting the underlying hepatic dysfunction. Normalization of hemodynamic parameters is observed after liver transplant [7].

To prevent severe hemodynamic decompensation in patients with cirrhosis, early identification and treatment of concomitant illnesses is important. Patients and parents are counseled on signs of intercurrent illness and on avoidance of hepatotoxic and cardiotoxic medication. Hypovolemia is to be avoided and rapidly treated in the case of gastroenteritis or febrile illness. A high index of suspicion for bacterial processes such as spontaneous peritonitis is warranted to initiate appropriate therapy without delay. Esophageal varices are monitored closely.

For the cirrhotic child requiring ICU admission for hemodynamic failure, high-output cardiac failure must be rapidly evaluated and treated. Volume repletion is commonly indicated, by crystalloid and by albumin replacement in hypoalbuminemic patients. Initial vasoactive treatment should address decreased systemic vascular resistance and usually includes norepinephrine in the absence of severe cardiomyopathy. Treatment is adjusted according to clinical and echocardiographic indices of cardiac output and vascular resistance.

Cirrhotic Cardiomyopathy

In advanced liver disease, hyperdynamic circulation gradually disappears as cardiac function and output decline with the onset of cirrhotic cardiomyopathy. This situation is less frequent in children as compared to adults.

Cirrhotic cardiomyopathy is characterized by systolic and diastolic ventricular dysfunction and by electrophysiological abnormalities, in the absence of underlying primary cardiac disease [8].

Though ventricular function tends to be preserved at rest, patients are at increased risk of hemodynamic decompensation in times of stress such as intercurrent illness. Pathophysiologic mechanisms include impaired beta-adrenergic signaling, altered cardiomyocyte cell membrane composition and ion channel defects, and increased endogenous cardiac inhibitory substances [9–11]. Cirrhotic cardiomyopathy is a risk factor for mortality and is reversible following liver transplant [12].

Pathophysiology

Impaired beta adrenergic signaling: In the setting of cirrhosis, impaired β-adrenergic signaling pathways result in decreased β-receptor density, decreased G-proteins, and decreased cAMP production, thus decreasing cardiac contractility by decreasing intracellular calcium influx.

Altered cardiomyocyte composition: The increased cholesterol content of cardiomyocyte cell wall may impair ion channel functioning.

Increased endogenous cardiac inhibitory substances in the cirrhotic patient include cannabinoids, which contribute to altered beta-adrenergic response, and NO and CO, which decrease intracellular calcium influx via excess c-GMP production.

Clinical Manifestations

The three principal manifestations of cirrhotic cardiomyopathy are systolic dysfunction, diastolic dysfunction, and electrophysiological anomalies.

Systolic dysfunction: Ventricular response to β-adrenergic inotropic and chronotropic stimuli is decreased due to downregulation of receptors and impaired signaling pathway. Left ventricular (LV) ejection fraction and cardiac output are often normal at rest, but do not increase in response to stress.

Diastolic dysfunction: The left ventricle is hypertrophied and noncompliant, with impaired relaxation and filling. The interventricular septum is thickened. On echocardiogram, impaired early diastolic (passive) filling by impaired ventricular relaxation is demonstrated by an E/A ratio <1. Clinical consequences of diastolic dysfunction include poor tolerance of tachycardia, hypovolemia, and anemia, and increased risk of certain arrhythmias such as atrial flutter.

Electrophysiological anomalies: Qtc interval prolongation, resulting from abnormal cardiac repolarization, is frequent, and is thought to be caused by functional changes in potassium channels in cardiac plasma membranes. This results in a delay between cardiac excitation and contraction. Length of Qtc interval is correlated with severity of hepatic disease, is partly reversible after β-blocker therapy, and normalizes after liver transplant. Despite the increased risk of ventricular arrhythmias with Qtc prolongation, these remain uncommon in patients with cirrhosis. The sinus node's ability to increase heart rate in response to increased oxygen demand is also impaired [13].

The onset of clinical manifestations of cirrhotic cardiomyopathy is latent. Left ventricular afterload is decreased by cirrhosis-induced systemic vasodilation, initially compensating for its decreasing systolic function. Diastolic dysfunction is also often asymptomatic at rest. Decompensation occurs in times of stress, when the cirrhotic heart is unable to increase output appropriately.

> Cirrhotic cardiomyopathy occurs less frequently in children than in adults, but its presence should be evaluated in patients with advanced cirrhosis, and considered in the cirrhotic child admitted to intensive care for hemodynamic compromise.

Treatment

Treatment of cirrhotic cardiomyopathy includes targeted hemodynamic therapy and early recognition and treatment of intercurrent illness. Recognition of chronotropic incompetence in the cirrhotic patient is important, as tachycardia is otherwise usually an early sign of infection and hemodynamic compromise in children.

Hemodynamic support targets the specific physiological abnormalities of cirrhotic cardiomyopathy: systolic and diastolic dysfunction and electrophysiological anomalies, as well as the peripheral arterial dilation of high-output cardiac failure. Beta-agonist inotropes (epinephrine, dobutamine), may be less effective due to receptor downregulation and impaired signaling. Echocardiography and cardiac output measures are useful to guide management.

Somewhat paradoxically, beta-blockers remain beneficial in the treatment of cirrhotic cardiomyopathy [14]. Aldosterone inhibitors may be useful [15]. In pediatric patients with cirrhotic cardiomyopathy, physiology normalizes after liver transplantation.

Hepatic Complications of Pediatric Cardiac Disease

Cardiac insufficiency is the heart's inability to provide sufficient blood flow and oxygen delivery to meet systemic needs. Cardiac insufficiency may result from decreased ventricular preload, increased ventricular afterload, arrhythmia, or primary ventricular systolic or diastolic dysfunction. The most common causes of primary cardiac insufficiency in young children are congenital structural abnormalities and cardiomyopathy; in older children acquired heart disease such as viral myocarditis becomes more likely, though cardiomyopathy may present at any age. Depending on the cause of cardiac dysfunction, symptom apparition may be rapid and severe, such as in myocarditis or severe left ventricular outflow tract obstruction upon closure of the ductus arteriosus, or more indolent, such as in dilated cardiomyopathy, which may not present until severe, or when compensatory mechanisms are overcome by an intercurrent infection.

A complete review of the etiology, diagnosis, and treatment of pediatric cardiac insufficiency is beyond the scope of this chapter. The hepatic consequences of cardiac insufficiency occur from ischemia due to inadequate oxygen delivery, and congestion from elevated central venous pressure. While hepatic dysfunction secondary to acute cardiac failure is reversible, repeated or chronic heart failure increases risk of hepatic fibrosis, cirrhosis, and hepatocellular carcinoma [16].

Hepatic Complications of Acute Cardiac Insufficiency: Ischemic Hepatitis

Ischemic hepatitis has many names: shock liver, acute cardiac liver, hypoxic liver, and post-shock hepatic failure. The *pathophysiology* of ischemic hepatitis is hypothesized to result from hepatic hypoxemia, reperfusion injury, reduced liver perfusion, hepatic congestion, and impaired hepatocellular oxygen uptake in the setting of severe low cardiac output state or acute circulatory failure mainly observed after septic or cardiogenic shock (dilated myocardiopathy or after cardiac surgery, for example) [17, 18]. This is seen when the strong defense mechanisms of the liver against anoxic injury are overcome.

Clinical exam reveals hepatomegaly and hepatalgia from rapid distention of the hepatic capsule. *Laboratory findings* include potentially massive elevation of transaminases coming from several tissues (muscles, red blood cells, liver) with aspartate aminotransferase (AST) levels above alanine aminotransferase (ALT) levels, and evidence of impaired synthetic function: prolonged International Normalized Ratio (INR), decreased factor VII, hypoalbuminemia, and hypoglycemia. Gamma-glutamyl transpeptidase (GGT), alkaline phosphatase (ALP), and bilirubin levels are less frequently perturbed, except in the context of preexisting chronic heart disease [19]. Typical *histological findings* are of centrilobular necrosis without immune cell infiltrate. *Treatment* is mainly supportive, and *prognosis* of ischemic hepatitis depends on the underlying etiology and reversibility of the shock state. Once hemodynamics are restored, the clinical and laboratory signs of ischemic hepatitis regress and normalize within 1 to 2 weeks [18].

Fontan-Associated Liver Disease (FALD)

The Fontan operation was first performed in 1968 as a palliation for tricuspid atresia. The original procedure has undergone modifications throughout the years and is currently the final procedure in staged palliation for a wide range of congenital heart lesions for which biventricular repair cannot be achieved. Based on the premise that central venous pressure can drive adequate preload to the single systemic ventricle when pulmonary vascular resistance is low, the goal of staged palliation to the Fontan is to volume unload the single systemic ventricle. The Fontan procedure also restores normal systemic arterial saturation to previously cyanotic patients.

Early and long-term survival of Fontan-palliated patients has improved significantly, with 30-year survival now near 85% [20]. It is estimated that 50–70,000 recipients of the procedure are alive today, with 40% above 18 years of age [21]. As increasing numbers of patients survive into adulthood, the long-term consequences of Fontan physiology on end organs, particularly the liver, are increasingly recognized. The 2017 American College of Cardiology Conference Report "Fontan-Associated Liver Disease" and the 2019 American Heart Association consensus guidelines on the "*Evaluation and Management of the Child and Adult with Fontan Circulation*" form the basis of this chapter [22, 23].

The Fontan circulation is unique in its absence of a subpulmonic ventricle. In order to relieve the volume load from two circulations to a single functioning ventricle, staged procedures isolate systemic venous return from the heart by anastomosing the superior vena cava (superior cavo-pulmonary connection) followed later by the inferior vena cava (total cavo-pulmonary connection), directly to the pulmonary artery [24]. The ventricular volume unloading and normal systemic arterial saturation provided by the Fontan procedure are at the cost of chronically elevated venous pressure and low cardiac output with preload restriction.

Cardiac insufficiency with venous congestion induces hepatic centrilobular congestion and inflammation [25]. With chronic exposure, hepatic fibrosis and cirrhosis develop, and repeated inflammatory hepatic insults are associated with increased incidence of hepatic carcinoma and hepatocellular adenoma [26].

Liver fibrosis and cirrhosis have been identified as early as 5 years postoperatively after the Fontan operation, and Fontan-associated liver disease (FALD) is a focus of increasing study as greater proportions of patients reach adulthood.

Pathophysiology

Profound changes in hepatic flow occur immediately after the Fontan surgery [23]: venous pressure acutely increases, cardiac output decreases, and lymphatic congestion occurs. Hepatic rigidity is seen early after surgery and persists. Elevated central venous pressure (CVP) is transmitted to the hepatic veins, sinusoids, and portal vein, thereby decreasing portal venous inflow. In response, hepatic arterial inflow increases above its usual 25% in order to maintain hepatic blood flow [27]. When CVP exceeds 20-25 mmHg, as during exercise or if there is Fontan pathway dysfunction, the hepatic buffer response cannot fully compensate for decreased portal vein inflow, and liver hypoperfusion occurs. Arterialized nodules are frequently found on follow-up of Fontan patients [28], but without direct correlation to the severity of FALD. The increased venous return resulting from arterialization of hepatic inflow is a recognized risk factor for hepatic fibrosis [29].

Clinical Presentation

Fontan-associated liver disease progresses insidiously and is long asymptomatic, apart from clinical hepatomegaly. Cirrhotic decompensations are rare, although some degree of fibrosis and compensated cirrhosis is present on liver histology. There is a poor correlation between liver imaging and histology, and with synthetic and detoxification functions. *Laboratory results* show a moderate elevation of ALT and AST without prognostic value. During remote monitoring, 84% of patients present at least one abnormal liver function test, the most common being an increase in GGT (70%) followed by an increase in total bilirubin. Increases in prothrombin time and the INR are observed [30]. Elevated venous pressures and splenic consumption cause thrombocytopenia. *Post-Fontan abdominal imaging* in adolescents and adults reveals a broad spectrum of abnormalities including heterogeneous liver, segmental enlargement or atrophy, irregular hepatic contours, splenomegaly, and ascites [31]. Ultrasound provides little information on the degree of fibrosis but provides structural information (hepatomegaly or splenomegaly, caudate lobe hypertrophy, for example), as well as hemodynamic information (anterograde portal venous flow, arterialization of hepatic flows, modification of mesenteric resistance). Computed tomography and MRI specify the morphology and structure of the liver and its vascularization [32]. Contrast-injected imaging is particularly useful for characterizing hepatic nodules. Hepatic stiffness is increasingly assessed with elastography, which appears to correlate with the degree of FALD [33] and is considered a valuable tool for assessing the progression of cirrhosis. MRI-coupled liver elastography combines both anatomical and stiffness data, providing a comprehensive assessment tool for FALD [34]. A wide spectrum of *histological abnormalities* are described with FALD, with varying degrees of fibrosis and cirrhosis [35]. These histological changes may be reversible following a heart transplant. One of the most serious hepatic manifestations of the Fontan circulation is the increased prevalence (1.3%) of hepatocellular carcinoma (HCC), at median age of 30 years old (range of 12–52 years old) [36]. The prognosis of HCC is poor with mortality greater than 50% 2 years after diagnosis. The prognosis is better when carcinoma is diagnosed in the asymptomatic phase. The association between an increased risk of carcinoma and FALD severity or cirrhosis is not clear, and remains to be studied.

Treatment

A primary and secondary prevention strategy for the liver must be implemented. Any rapid change in hepatic parameters should warrant a thorough hemodynamic evaluation to evaluate valvular sufficiency, Fontan or aortic arch obstruction, ventricular systolic or diastolic dysfunction, pulmonary vascular disease, or arrhythmia, with intervention as necessary. Surgical innovations, such as the exclusion of the hepatic vein, have a short-term beneficial effect, but have not been demonstrated to be effective in the long term and include complications such as worsening cyanosis. The use of pulmonary vasodilators, diuretics, antifibrotics (aldosterone inhibitors), and angiotensin converting enzyme (ACE) inhibitors have theoretical benefit. In practice, they do not prevent the development of FALD. Hepatic prevention medicine is recommended for all Fontan patients: avoidance of drugs and hepatotoxic substances (acetaminophen, alcohol) and vaccination against hepatitis B are recommended.

> Patients with a Fontan circulation must have regular monitoring with a multidisciplinary team including (but not restricted to) cardiologist, hepatologist, and cardiac surgeon in a tertiary care setting.

Conclusion

The liver is a "venous reservoir" and metabolic factory in close proximity to the heart; its examination provides critical information on a child's hemodynamic status. Heart failure directly impacts liver function, and hepatic dysfunction has significant hemodynamic consequences. The management of cirrhotic patients during cardiac decompensation is challenging and requires an appreciation for the complex interdependence between the liver and the heart. Improved long-term survival of patients with congenital heart disease, and specifically with the Fontan circulation, has given rise to new and complex liver disease.

References

1. Schrier RW, Arroyo V, Bernardi M, Epstein M, Henriksen JH, Rode's J. Peripheral arterial vasodilation hypothesis : a proposal for the initiation of renal sodium and water retention in cirrhosis. Hepatology. 1988;8:1151–7.
2. Vallance P, Moncada S. Hyperdynamic circulation in cirrhosis: a role for nitric oxide? Lancet. 1991;337:776–8.
3. Møller S, Henriksen JH. Cardiovascular complications of cirrhosis. Gut. 2008;57:268–78.
4. Sanyal AJ, Boyer TD, Lindor KD, Terrault NA. Zakim and Boyer's hepatology: a textbook of liver disease. 7th ed. Philadelphia: Elsevier; 2018.
5. Martin PY, Ginès P, Schrier RW. Nitric oxide as a mediator of hemodynamic abnormalities and sodium and water retention in cirrhosis. N Engl J Med. 1998;339:533.
6. Abraldes JG, Iwakiri Y, Loureiro-Silva M, Haq O, Sessa WC, Groszmann RJ. Mild increases in portal pressure up-regulate VEGF and eNOS in the intestinal microcirculation leading to hyperdynamic state. Am J Physiol Gastrointest Liver Physiol. 2006;290:980.
7. Vaughan RB, Angus PW, Chin-Dusting JP. Evidence for altered vascular responses to exogenous endothelin-1 in patients with advanced cirrhosis with restoration of the normal vasoconstrictor response following successful liver transplantation. Gut. 2004;53:470–1.
8. Ma Z, Lee SS. Cirrhotic cardiomyopathy : getting to the heart of the matter. Hepatology. 1996;24:451–9.
9. Páll A, Czifra A, Vitális S, Papp M, Paragh G, Szabó Z. Pathophysiological and clinical approach to cirrhotic cardiomyopathy. J Gastrointestin Liver Dis. 2014;23:301–10.
10. Lee RF, Glenn TK, Lee SS. Cardiac dysfunction in cirrhosis. Best Pract Res Clin Gastroenterol. 2007;21:125–40.
11. Seirafi M, Spahr L. La cardiomyopathie cirrhotique. Rev Med Suisse. 2009;5:1725–31.
12. Torregrosa M, Aguadé S, Dos L, et al. Cardiac alterations in cirrhosis : reversibility after liver transplantation. J Hepatol. 2005;42:68–74.
13. Genovesi S, Prata Pizzala DM, Pozzi M, et al. QT interval prolongation and decreased heart rate variability in cirrhotic patients : relevance of hepatic venous pressure gradient and serum calcium. Clin Sci. 2009;116:851–9.
14. Zambruni A, et al. Effects of chronic beta-blockade interval in patients with liver cirrhosis. J Hepatol. 2008;48:415–21.
15. Pozzi M, Grassi G, Ratti L, et al. Cardiac, neuroadrenergic, and portal hemodynamic effects of prolonged aldosterone blockade in post-viral child a cirrhosis. Am J Gastroenterol. 2005;100:1110–6.
16. Liver disease secondary to congenital heart disease in children. Expert Rev Gastroenterol Hepatol. 2019;13:651–66.

17. Valla DC. Hypoxie hépatique, foie cardiaque congestif. Gastroenterol Clin Biol. 2003;27(sup 5):33–40.
18. Waseem M, Chen PH. Hypoxic hepatitis : a review and clinical update. J Clin Transl Hepatol. 2016;4:263–8.
19. Birgens HS, Henriksen J, Matzen P, Poulsen H. The shock liver. Clinical and biochemical findings in patients with centrilobular liver necrosis following cardiogenic shock. Acta Med Scand. 1978;204:417–21.
20. Pundi KN, Johnson JN, Dearani JA, Pundi KN, Li Z, Hinck CA, Dahl SH, Cannon BC, O'Leary PW, Driscoll DJ, Cetta F. 40-year follow-up after the Fontan operation: long-term outcomes of 1,052 patients. J Am Coll Cardiol. 2015;66:1700–10.
21. Schilling C, Dalziel K, Nunn R, Du Plessis K, Shi WY, Celermajer D, Winlaw D, Weintraub RG, Grigg LE, Radford DJ, Bullock A, Gentles TL, Wheaton GR, Hornung T, Justo RN, d'Udekem Y. The Fontan epidemic : population projections from the Australia and New Zealand Fontan Registry. Int J Cardiol. 2016;219:14–9.
22. Rychik J, Atz AM, Celermajer DS, Deal BJ, Gatzoulis MA, Gewillig MH, Hsia TY, Hsu DT, Kovacs AH, McCrindle BW, Newburger JW, Pike NA, Rodefeld M, Rosenthal DN, Schumacher KR, Marino BS, Stout K, Veldtman G, Younoszai AK, d'Udekem Y, American Heart Association Council on Cardiovascular Disease in the Young and Council on Cardiovascular and Stroke Nursing. Evaluation and management of the child and adult with Fontan circulation. A scientific statement from the American Heart Association. Circulation. 2019;140:e234–84.
23. Daniels CJ, Bradley EA, Landzberg MJ, Aboulhosn J, Beekman RH, Book W, Gurvitz M, John A, John B, Marelli A, Marino BS, Minich LL, Poterucha JJ, Rand EB, Veldtman GR. Fontan-associated liver disease: proceedings from the American College of Cardiology Stakeholders Meeting, October 1 to 2, 2015, Washington DC. J Am Coll Cardiol. 2017;70:3173–94.
24. Gewillig M, Brown SC. The Fontan circulation after 45 years: update in physiology. Heart. 2016;102:1081–6.
25. Arcidi JM Jr, Moore GW, Hutchins GM. Hepatic morphology in cardiac dysfunction: a clinicopathologic study of 1000 subjects at autopsy. Am J Pathol. 1981;104:159–66.
26. Ghaferi AA, Hutchins GM. Progression of liver pathology in patients undergoing the Fontan procedure: chronic passive congestion, cardiac cirrhosis, hepatic adenoma, and hepatocellular carcinoma. J Thorac Cardiovasc Surg. 2005;129:1348–52.
27. Lautt WW, Legare DJ, d'Almeida MS. Adenosine as putative regulator of hepatic arterial flow (the buffer response). Am J Phys. 1985;248:H331–8.
28. Bryant T, Ahmad Z, Millward-Sadler H, Burney K, Stedman B, Kendall T, Vettukattil J, Haw M, Salmon AP, Cope R, Hacking N, Breen D, Sheron N, Veldtman GR. Arterialised hepatic nodules in the Fontan circulation : hepatico-cardiac interactions. Int J Cardiol. 2011;151:268–72.
29. Trusty PM, Wei Z, Rychik J, Russo PA, Surrey LF, Goldberg DJ, Fogel MA, Yoganathan AP. Impact of hemodynamics and fluid energetics on liver fibrosis after Fontan operation. J Thorac Cardiovasc Surg. 2018;156:267–75.
30. van Nieuwenhuizen RC, Peters M, Lubbers LJ, Trip MD, Tijssen JG, Mulder BJ. Abnormalities in liver function and coagulation profile following the Fontan procedure. Heart. 1999;82:40–6.
31. Wu FM, Kogon B, Earing MG, Aboulhosn JA, Broberg CS, John AS, Harmon A, Sainani NI, Hill AJ, Odze RD, Johncilla ME, Ukomadu C, Gauvreau K, Valente AM, Landzberg MJ. Alliance for adult research in congenital cardiology (AARCC) investigators. Liver health in adults with Fontan circulation: a multicenter cross-sectional study. J Thorac Cardiovasc Surg. 2017;153:656–64.
32. Hilscher MB, Johnson JN, Cetta F, Driscoll DJ, Poterucha JJ, Sanchez W, Connolly HM, Kamath PS. Surveillance for liver complications after the Fontan procedure. Congenit Heart Dis. 2017;12:124–32.
33. Chen B, Schreiber RA, Human DG, Potts JE, Guttman OR. Assessment of liver stiffness in pediatric Fontan patients using transient elastography. Can J Gastroenterol Hepatol. 2016;2016:7125193.

34. Poterucha JT, Johnson JN, Qureshi MY, O'Leary PW, Kamath PS, Lennon RJ, Bonnichsen CR, Young PM, Venkatesh SK, Ehman RL, Gupta S, Smyrk TC, Dearani JA, Warnes CA, Cetta F. Magnetic resonance elastography: a novel technique for the detection of hepatic fibrosis and hepatocellular carcinoma after the Fontan operation. Mayo Clin Proc. 2015;90:882–94.
35. Goldberg DJ, Surrey LF, Glatz AC, Dodds K, O'Byrne ML, Lin HC, Fogel M, Rome JJ, Rand EB, Russo P, Rychik J. Hepatic fibrosis is universal following Fontan operation, and severity is associated with time from surgery: a liver biopsy and hemodynamic study. J Am Heart Assoc. 2017;6:e004809.
36. Egbe AC, Poterucha JT, Warnes CA, Connolly HM, Baskar S, Ginde S, Clift P, Kogon B, Book WM, Walker N, Wagenaar L, Moe T, Oechslin E, Kay WA, Norris M, Gordon-Walker T, Dillman JR, Trout A, Anwar N, Hoskoppal A, Veldtman GR. Hepatocellular carcinoma after Fontan operation. Circulation. 2018;138:746–8.

Liver Failure and Haematopoietic Stem Cell Transplantation

Laurence Tabone, Pierre Teira, and Annie Lavoie

Introduction

Approximately 17% to 35% of children undergoing stem cell transplantation (HSCT) will be admitted to the paediatric intensive care unit (PICU) [1]. Over the last 20 years, advances in the field of HSCT have decreased the transplantation related morbidity and mortality and improved the overall outcome of HSCT [2, 3]. Even if mortality of post-HSCT children admitted to PICU has also decreased, their risk of death is still high [4]. Taking in charge post-HSCT children in PICU requires to understand the multiple and complex physiopathologies of organ toxicities encountered in the first weeks after HSCT. Among possible organ toxicities, the liver is at high risk of injury during HSCT. Liver damages may come from the underlying pathology, previous medications and complications before HSCT, as well as from direct toxicity of conditioning regimen, infection prophylaxis and treatment, prolonged parenteral nutrition, sepsis, viral infections, systemic endothelial diseases including graft vs. host disease (GVHd), transplant-associated microangiopathy and sinusoidal obstructive syndrome (SOS). SOS, formerly known as

L. Tabone
Pediatric Intensive Care Unit, Department of Pediatrics, CHU Sainte-Justine, Université de Montréal, Montreal, QC, Canada
e-mail: laurence.tabone.med@ssss.gouv.qc.ca

P. Teira (✉)
Hematology-Oncology Unit, Department of Pediatrics, CHU Sainte-Justine, Université de Montréal, Montreal, QC, Canada
e-mail: pierre.teira.med@ssss.gouv.qc.ca

A. Lavoie
Department of Pharmacist, CHU Sainte-Justine, Université de Montréal, Montreal, QC, Canada
e-mail: annie.lavoie.hsj@ssss.gouv.qc.ca

P. Jouvet, F. Alvarez (eds.), *Liver Diseases in the Pediatric Intensive Care Unit*,
https://doi.org/10.1007/978-3-030-79132-2_9

hepatic veno-occlusive disease (VOD), is a common cause of admission to PICU with a 50% risk of death for severe forms [5]. Other causes of liver damages are also discussed in this chapter, although they are not generally responsible for admission in intensive care per se. Finally, potentially hepatotoxic treatments and therapeutic adjustments will be discussed in a separate section.

Sinusoidal Obstructive Syndrome

Sinusoidal obstructive syndrome (SOS) is the most frequent liver injury in children undergoing HSCT. It affects 22% to 30% of children after HSCT and up to 60% in high-risk populations [6]. Progression to multiple organ failure (MOF) occurs in 30% to 60% of cases. Occasionally, SOS has also been reported, outside of HSCT, in children treated with actinomycine, cyclophosphamide or abdominal radiotherapy for Wilms' tumours, rhabdomyosarcomas and rare brain tumours. Former studies were based on diagnostic criteria established on adult data. Due to paediatric specificities of the clinical presentation, diagnostic criteria in children have been recently redefined (see below) [6, 7].

Even if SOS had not been associated with PICU mortality in recent studies, it can lead to multiple organ dysfunction syndrome and necessitates support. SOS leading to MOF constitutes independent mortality factors in PICU [1]. Key of management is early recognition and aggressive treatment before occurrence of MOF [7–10].

Physiopathology

The primary step to SOS is sinusoidal endothelial cell damage triggered by multiple injuries such as toxicity of the conditioning regimen, pro-inflammatory cytokines, infections and medications. Once the endothelial cells are damaged, they become rounder and the sinus barrier is disrupted. Gaps in the sinusoidal barrier allow the accumulation of cellular debris in the space of Disse beneath the endothelial cells, participating in the obstruction of sinusoidal vessels. The damage of the endothelial barrier trigger the activation of thrombosis, platelets deposit and clot formation in the sinusoidal vessels contributing to the obstruction. Finally, hepatocytes dysfunction related to alteration of glutathione enzymatic system and accumulation of toxic metabolites may aggravate the phenomenon as well as large amounts of reactive oxidation species due to iron overload and radiotherapy.

Endothelial damage leads to capillary leak syndrome, driving to ascites, pleural effusion and generalized oedema. Portal hypertension and high daily fluid intakes aggravate the phenomenon. Resulting fluid overload can contribute to acute respiratory failure. Moreover, hepatic injuries of SOS can result in hepatocellular necrosis and liver failure. Acute kidney injury can result from abdominal compartment syndrome, intravascular volume depletion or hepato-renal syndrome.

Risk Factors of SOS

Precise identification of high-risk patients is necessary both to identify patients requiring specific prophylaxis but also to improve the prognosis by establishing an early treatment [11]. Risk factors can be classified into two categories: patient-related factors and transplantation-related factors. They are summarized in Table 1. Patient-related factors include age under 2 years old [12], female gender, genetic predisposition [13, 14], pre-existing liver disease and specific indications for HSCT such as osteopetrosis, haemophagocytic lymphohistiocytosis [12], high-risk neuroblastoma, thalassemia and leukaemia beyond second relapse. Transplantation-related factors include myeloablative conditioning (MAC), early neutrophil engraftment, melphalan or busulfan conditioning especially in association with cyclophosphamide, sepsis post-HSCT and GVHD prophylaxis with sirolimus [15]. Furthermore, monoclonal antibodies (Ab) tagged with calicheamicin derivatives, such as gemtuzumab ozogamicin and inotuzumab ozogamicin used for treatment of acute myeloid leukaemia and acute lymphoblastic leukaemia, respectively, are risk factors of SOS/VOD, and onset can occur after Ab administration alone or in subsequent HSCT [16–18]. The higher incidence of SOS after HSCT is observed in children suffering from osteopetrosis where the risk is more than 50% [19].

> Recognition of predisposing factors for sinusoidal obstructive syndrome, leads to establish an early treatment to diminish morbidity and mortality associated with this complication.

Clinical Presentation and Diagnosis Criteria

The modified Seattle criteria and the Baltimore criteria were used for the diagnosis of SOS, both in adults and children. However, there are major differences between the two populations in terms of incidence, risk factors (age and underlying

Table 1 Reported risk factors associated with sinusoidal obstructive syndrome in children

Risk factors	
Patient-related factors	Transplantation-related factors
Genetic factors	Previous HSCT
Female gender	Prior treatment with gemtuzumab ozogamicin
Age < 2 years	Allogeneic versus autologous stem cell transplantation
Pre-existing liver disease	HLA mismatch
Underlying disease:	Conditioning regimen
HLH	Sepsis post HSCT
Osteopetrosis	GVHD prophylaxis
Thalassemia	Non-T cell-depleted grafts
Ferritin level > 1000 ng/mL	Acute hepatic/gut GVHD

diseases), clinical presentation and response to defibrotide [6]. Hence, in children, late-onset SOS can occur more than 30 days after transplantation and children can be anicteric in 30% of the cases [20]. The European Society for Blood and Marrow Transplantation (EBMT) has proposed new diagnostic criteria [6], taken up and developed by a recent international position statement from the Pediatric Acute Lung Injury and Sepsis Investigators (PALISI) Network and the Pediatric Diseases Working Party of the EBMT [7]. Thus, SOS in children is defined by the presence of two or more criteria among the following: unexplained consumptive and transfusion-refractory thrombocytopenia, otherwise unexplained weight gain on three consecutive days despite the use of diuretics or a weight gain >5% above baseline value, hepatomegaly, ascites, rising bilirubin from a baseline value on 3 consecutive days or bilirubin ≥2 mg/dL (34 μmol/L) within 72 h. The EBMT states there is no limitation of delay for onset of SOS. Hepatic doppler ultrasound (US) is not required for diagnosis, but in high-risk patients, a pre-transplant US should be used as a reference [8]. Once the diagnosis has been made, US can be useful to quantify ascites. Liver biopsy, portal venous wedge pressure and reversal of portal venous flow on doppler should not be used for the routine diagnosis of SOS. Clinical criteria are summarized in Table 2.

The peak of incidence for SOS diagnosis occurs for 70–80% of patients in the second or third week after infusion of the new bone marrow, with a large range reported between 1 to 104 day post HSCT [12].

Consumptive and transfusion-refractory thrombocytopenia should be seen as an early warning sign. The definition of platelet refractoriness varies according to the authors [6, 7] but can be defined simply as unexplained consumptive and transfusion refractory thrombocytopenia as at least one weight-adjusted platelet transfusion per day to maintain institutional guidelines. Platelet transfusions refractoriness may be encountered in another post-HSCT complication like thrombotic microangiopathy (TMA), but its association with high LDH blood level, high blood pressure and acute renal dysfunction with proteinuria help to diagnose TMA.

Growing hepatomegaly with or without exquisite pain in the upper right abdomen (hepatalgia) is often blurred by diffuse abdominal pain related to gut mucositis during the first 3 weeks after transplantation or by hepatomegaly due to the primary disease such as osteopetrosis, liver infiltration by leukaemia cells, thalassemia or

Table 2 Diagnostic criteria of the European Society for Blood and Marrow Transplantation for hepatic sinusoidal obstructive syndrome (SOS) in children

1. No limitation for time of onset of SOS
2. The presence of two or more of the following:
Unexplained consumptive and transfusion-refractory thrombocytopenia
Otherwise unexplained weight gain on 3 consecutive days despite the use of diuretics or a weight gain >5% above baseline value
Hepatomegaly above baseline value
Ascites above baseline value
Rising bilirubin from a baseline value on 3 consecutive days or bilirubin ≥2 mg/dL (34 micromol/L) within 72 h

mucopolysaccharidosis. To improve sensibility and specificity of clinical examination, it is recommended to perform a baseline abdominal ultrasound and to repeat it in case of suspicion of SOS [6, 7].

Weight gain related to fluid overload is also an early symptom and often evolves rapidly despite escalating dosing of diuretics. Daily or twice daily monitoring of weight gain is mandatory after HSCT. Fluid overload and weight gain may worsen within few days to massive ascites and hepato-renal syndrome. Then, pulmonary restrictive syndrome secondary to pleural effusion, massive hepatomegaly with hepatalgia and ascites leads to acute respiratory distress syndrome.

Bilirubin increase is usually late in disease evolution and is made of conjugated bilirubin predominantly. Once drug toxicity, infectious complication or liver acute graft versus host disease has been excluded, the increase in alanine amino-transferase (ALT) and asparagine amino-transferase (AST) is indicative of hepatic damage and is a severity criteria (Table 3). Thus, contrary to SOS presentation in adults, the absence of liver tests abnormalities should not make the diagnosis of SOS less likely in children.

Regarding radiology, reverse flow of portal vein is usually absent in early evolution of SOS. If reverse flow is noted on ultrasound doppler, the differential diagnosis of Budd Chiari syndrome has to be ruled out by the radiologist. Thickening and swelling of the gallbladder wall is a frequent ultrasound finding noted in SOS.

Once the diagnosis of SOS has been made, severity criteria are used to adjust the treatment and monitor its progress. SOS severity criteria defined by the EBMT [6] and secondary modified [7] are reported in Table 3.

Transfusion-refractory thrombocytopenia, unexplained weight gain, hepatomegaly, ascites and rising bilirubin are the main signs of sinusoidal obstructive syndrome.

Prevention

Prevention is based on supportive care and specific medications.

Patients undergoing HSCT, even in the absence of SOS, are at risk of fluid overload for two main reasons: conditioning regimen responsible for capillary leak syndrome and significant increase of daily fluid intake related to numerous medications, transfusions and parenteral nutrition. They should have aggressive fluid management because fluid overload increases the risk of PICU admission in children and increases mortality in adults [21, 22]. Fluid management is based on twice-daily weight monitoring, strict daily fluid balance calculation, use of maximized concentration of medications and parenteral nutrition [9].

Ursodeoxycholic acid (UA) is recommended for SOS prophylaxis [7, 8, 23] in children at risk: myelo-ablative conditioning based on high doses of chemotherapy with busulfan, melphalan and cyclophosphamide, previous use of mAb conjugated

Table 3 Severity grading thresholds of sinusoidal obstructive syndrome among children, adolescent and young adults

	Modified European Society for Blood and Marrow Transplantation severity grading			
	Mild	Moderate	Severe	Very severe
ALT, AST, GLDH (mg/dL)	<ou = 2 × normal	2–5 × normal	2–5 × normal	>5 × normal
Bilirubin (mg/dL)	<2	<2	≥2	Bilirubin doubles in 48 h
Coagulopathy: INR (not responding to vitamin K)	>1.5	1.5–1.9	>2	Need for replacement of coagulation factors
Ascites	Mild	Moderate	Severe	Requires paracentesis
Weight gain (from baseline)	2–5%	5–10% despite diuretic use	>10%	Persistent rise
Renal function score	KDIGO 1: serum creatinine 1.5–1.9 × baseline or ≥0.3 mg/dL (≥26.5 mmol/L) increase or urine output<0.5 mL/kg/h for 6–12 h	KDIGO 2 serum creatinine 2.0–2.9 × baseline or urine output<0.5 mL/kg/h for ≥12 h	KDIGO 3: serum creatinine 4.0 × baseline or ≥0.3 mg/dL (≥353.6 mmol/L) increase or urine output<0.3 mL/kg/h for ≥24 h or anuria for ≥12 h or initiation of RRT	Persistent need for renal replacement therapy
Encephalopathy	CADP <9	CADP <9	CADP ≥9	CADP ≥9
Persistent RT	<3 days	3–7 days	–	>7 days
Pulmonary function	<2 L	<2 L	NIV/IMV	IMV

ALT alanine aminotransferase, *AST* aspartate aminotransferase, *GLDH* glutamate dehydrogenase, *INR* international normalized ratio, *KDIGO* Kidney Disease: Improving Global Outcomes score, *RRT* renal replacement therapy, *CADP* Cornell Assessment of Pediatric Delirium, *RT* refractory thrombocytopenia, *NIV* non-invasive ventilation, *IMV* invasive mechanical ventilation

with calicheamicin drugs, hepatic dysfunction or damages present before HSCT and osteopetrosis. Ursodeoxycholic acid is a naturally occurring hydrophilic bile acid. As a nontoxic bile acid, ursodiol possibly reduces liver injury by replacement of endogenous bile acids that are more toxic. It can also have modulating effects on cytokine expression and anti-inflammatory effects. It has been shown to decrease the risk of developing SOS and to reduce all-cause mortality at 100 days after HSCT.

Defibrotide might be used, if feasible, for patients with high risk of SOS such as children and adolescent with osteopetrosis, familial haemophagocytic lymphohistiocytosis, second MAC transplantation, previous treatment with calicheamicin-bound conjugated drug, high-risk neuroblastoma, thalassemia and all infants undergoing HSCT [7, 23]. Defibrotide appears to attenuate endothelial cell activation and protect endothelial cells from inflammation and prothrombotic state that is generated by their activation. It promotes the enzymatic action of plasmin, thus increasing fibrinolysis, restoring the thrombo-fibrinolytic balance and improving hepatic microvascular circulation. Despite its antithrombotic action, it is not associated with significant bleeding risk.

Due to this lack of solid evidence of prophylactic efficacy and to its high tag price also, defibrotide prophylaxis tends to be restricted to very high-risk patients only.

Heparin, low-molecular-weight heparins (LMWH), fresh frozen plasma (FFP), antithrombin III, glutamine or prostaglandin E1 are not recommended for SOS prophylaxis because of lack of evidence [8].

Prevention is reserved for patients with known factors predisposing to sinusoidal obstructive syndrome.

Treatment

Mild and moderate forms can be managed by supportive care in association with very close monitoring of disease evolution, mainly through daily or twice daily routine clinical exam. Specific early medication with defibrotide is recommended for patients with severe SOS or moderate SOS progressing under supportive care. Dose regimen is 25 mg/kg divided into 4 daily doses intravenously with a duration of 21 days or until resolution of SOS signs [7, 8]. Doses up to 40 mg/kg and 60 mg/kg daily have been tested in adults with very severe forms, but this higher dose was not more effective and was associated with higher risk of bleeding. The EBMT recommends prompt defibrotide use without consideration of severity grade or organ damage [23]. This recommendation is based on the observation that defibrotide appears less effective if initiated late in the course of SOS after multiple organ failures develop. The mechanisms of action of defibrotide are multiple. It is believed to reduce the activation of endothelial cells and protect them from toxic, inflammatory, and reperfusion damage. In addition, it helps to restore the thrombo-fibrinolytic balance [24]. Of note, defibrotide is not an anticoagulation therapy and does not increase the risk of bleeding at the standard dose of 25 mg/kg. Defibrotide represents a breakthrough for SOS treatment and the incidence of fatal SOS has dramatically decreased since its use. The exact duration of defibrotide treatment has not been established and is mainly based on the resolution of symptoms, which can take 2 to 4 weeks. Early discontinuation of defibrotide after the first signs of clinical and biologic improvement may be followed by SOS worsening.

For patient progressing on defibrotide treatment and best supportive care, although non-recommended, corticosteroids bolus (methylprednisolone 500 mg/m^2 per dose every 12 h for 6 doses) could be considered. Preliminary positive results still need to be confirmed through a randomized trial. In a situation of rapidly evolving SOS despite defibrotide, given the lack of other options and the known toxicity profile of methylprednisolone bolus, this option may be considered.

Supportive care in these patients is based on aggressive fluid management, ventilatory, haemodynamic and transfusion support. Due to the risk of haemorrhage and infection, any invasive procedure must be carefully considered. Criteria for intensive care hospitalization are not described in the recommendations, but any severe or moderate form that progresses rapidly should lead to the paediatric intensive care unit admission.

Fluids Management

Fluid management is essential in symptomatic treatment of SOS. The aim is to achieve patient's baseline weight with fluids restriction (total fluid intake up to 50–75% of maintenance fluid requirements), diuretics and albumin (if serum albumin<3 g/dL). Figure 1 is presenting an algorithm for fluid overload management in SOS [9]. Fluid restriction may be problematic in severe forms of SOS, especially for kidney tolerance of immunosuppressive medications (ciclosporin, tacrolimus or sirolimus) or antiviral therapy (acyclovir, foscavir, cidofovir).

In case of persistent ascites despite well-conducted medical treatment, especially if it is responsible for abdominal compartment syndrome or respiratory failure, paracentesis should be considered. Paracentesis is usually at limited risk of bleeding

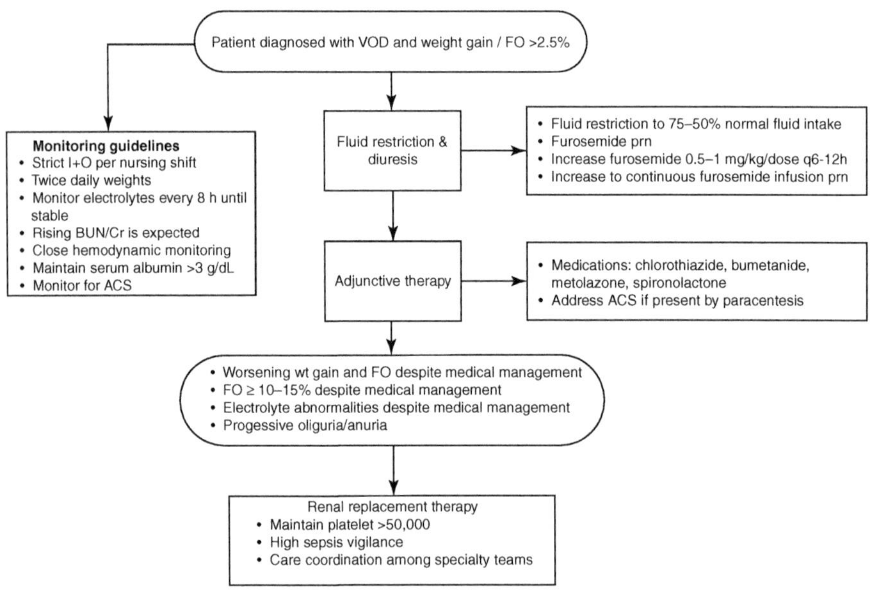

Fig. 1 Flow sheet for various interventions in a patient with veno-occlusive disease (VOD). FO fluid overload, ACS abdominal compartment syndrome, PRN as needed, I + O: intake and output (Reproduced from Mahadeo et al. [9])

even in case of low platelet counts despite daily or twice daily transfusion. The main risk is of large fluid loss, followed by hypovolemic shock, after insertion of the peritoneal catheter, due to the high concentration of albumin and the rapid reformation of ascites. This risk is easily manageable by limiting the drainage flow at a maximal initial rate of 5 mL/kg/hour. Infusion of albumin (0.5 to 1 g/kg) can be used to correct hypoalbuminemia following paracentesis. It is recommended to clamp the peritoneal drain for 24 h if drainage is <5 mL/kg/day. In the absence of recurrent signs of respiratory failure, abdominal discomfort, or reaccumulating ascites, the drain is removed [9].

Thoracocentesis has to be considered in case of pleural effusions responsible for poor oxygenation and ventilation. Because of the risk of expansion, pulmonary oedema and hypotension, no more than 10 mL/kg should be removed in the first hour. When the drainage is <3 mL/kg/day, chest drains could be removed after 24 h of clamping. Of note, paracentesis is often effective to drain pleural effusion in children and permits to avoid thoracocentesis.

Because of the risk of bleeding, infection and hypotension in these patients, indication for continuous renal therapy replacement (CRRT) should be carefully assessed. CRRT should be considered in case of worsening fluid overload, electrolyte abnormalities and progressive oliguria or anuria, despite optimal medical management. To minimize risk of bleeding, regional citrate should be preferred for circuit anticoagulation, in the absence of severe liver failure. Threshold of platelet transfusions should be discussed on a case-per-case basis in this situation. While a target of more than 30 or 50 $x10^9/l$ may be recommended to reduce the risk of bleeding related to CRRT, it is often impossible to achieve during severe SOS. Moreover, massive platelets transfusion is at risk of SOS worsening. Calcineurin inhibitors are at risk of overdosing during SOS, since 90% of ciclosporin and tacrolimus metabolites elimination is done by the liver. Cholestasis leads to intoxication by calcineurin inhibitors, which in turn increases kidney damages and worsen hepato-renal syndrome. Thus these medications should be decreased or discontinued and changed to GVHD prophylaxis based on methylprednisolone or mycophenolate mofetil.

Transfusion Support

Current recommendations have set a platelet transfusion threshold of $20x10^9$ for patients not on thrombolytic therapy and a threshold of $30x10^9$ for patients on thrombolytic therapy, including patients on defibrotide [9]. However, these recommendations should be adapted to each situation: repeated platelet transfusions may worsen the SOS and these thresholds may be impossible to reach when there is major platelet consumption. Cryoprecipitate, tranexamic acid and frozen plasma are not recommended in the absence of bleeding.

Red Blood Cells (RBC) low-dose transfusion (10 to 15 mL/kg) is recommended for haemoglobin levels under 70 g/L, as for every patient post HSCT [25]. Higher threshold of RBC transfusions (more than 100 g/L) has been associated with the onset of severe SOS in a randomized study on RBC transfusions [26].

In case of acute bleeding, defibrotide should be discontinued. Blood products (fresh frozen plasma, cryoprecipitate, platelets) and vitamin K can be guided by the use of viscoelastic monitoring devices. Data are limited on the use of recombinant activated factor VII.

Ventilation

Significant ascites, pleural effusions and hepatomegaly are responsible for restrictive respiratory failure and atelectasis. Hypoventilation related to accumulation of sedative and opioid drugs can aggravate the process. Pulmonary interstitial oedema related to capillary leakage and fluid overload alters oxygenation. At last, damage to the pulmonary small veins and venules may occur in the context of SOS leading to rare cases of lung veno-occlusive disease.

Data are lacking to recommend non-invasive ventilation (NIV) or high-flow nasal cannula, but in cases of severe hypoxia, impaired alertness or upper airway obstruction, intubation is indicated [10]. Lung-protective strategy according to the Pediatric Acute Lung Injury Consensus Conference Group should be used [27], with a tidal volume calculated on dry weight given the almost constant fluids overload at this stage of management. It should be noted that in these patients, due to the conditions described above, chest compliance is often decreased, protecting the lung and allowing to tolerate higher inspiratory pressures, up to 32 cm H_2O [10, 27].

There is no evidence on the optimum use of high-frequency oscillatory ventilation (HFOV) in children with SOS.

There are no data on the use of ECMO in children presenting SOS plus ARDS and no recommendation could be made [10]. However, mortality rate of children undergoing ECMO post HSCT is about 80% [28, 29].

Nutrition

Prevention of gastrointestinal bleeding by a proton pump inhibitor is recommended for all patients with SOS. Whenever possible, enteral nutrition should be preferred to parenteral nutrition to maximize control of fluid overload and to maintain entero-hepatic circulation of biliary salts for prevention and eventual treatment of cholestasis.

Infection Treatments

There is no infectious surveillance nor antibio-prophylaxis required in addition to the recommended post-HSCT surveillance [10]. But one of the leading cause of death at day +100 post HSCT in adult and children remains infection [30]. Any fever should lead to prophylactic antibiotic therapy. Any aggravation of cholestasis is not necessarily related to SOS but may also be due to sepsis.

Particular attention must be paid to the risk of fungal infection: several cases of aspergillus and candida infections mimicking SOS have been reported, furthermore the presence of a fungal infection prior to HSCT is associated with a four-fold risk of developing SOS, and finally antifungal medications prophylaxis is often suspended during the period of SOS, because of hepatotoxicity. Thus, weekly monitoring of serum galactomannan may be considered for patients with SOS. Prompt initiation of treatment preferentially based on amphotericin B (Ambisome[R]) or echinocandins should be discussed when fungal infections are suspected.

Even in the context of SOS, any alteration in liver function tests can be due to a hepatotropic virus, and lead to viral testing using polymerase chain reaction for detection of cytomegalovirus, Epstein-Barr virus, human herpesvirus 6, adenovirus, herpes simplex virus and varicella zoster virus [10].

Non-specific intravenous immunoglobulins are not recommended [10] as no study has shown a benefit [31].

Liver Dysfunction Treatment

SOS can lead to fulminant hepatic failure (FHF) defined by hepatic encephalopathy (HE) and severe liver dysfunction. Recommended treatment of FHF is not specific. Even if data on their use in this cause of FHF are lacking, lactulose and rifaximin are recommended to decrease the uptake of glutamine and ammonia in the intestine. Intracranial pression should be monitored by transcranial Doppler ultrasound. Common measures to reduce intracranial pressure include minimizing patient agitation and stimulation, elevating the head of patient's bed and optimizing sodium serum levels between 145 and 155 mEq/L. Also, normocapnia and normoxia must be maintained if the patient is ventilated, and hypoglycaemia corrected.

Liver transplantation may be considered for some patients with fulminant SOS with FHF without relapse of the original disease. Good prognosis after HSCT is recorded, if there is an effective bone marrow engraftment, no GVHd, no active infection and no severe failure of another organ [10]. Only a few paediatric liver transplant cases have been reported in the context of fulminant SOS [32, 33].

Delirium Treatment

Routine screening for delirium is recommended with the Cornell Assessment of Pediatric Delirium (CAPD) or the Pediatric Confusion Assessment Method for the ICU (pCAM-ICU), given that children undergoing HSCT cumulate risk factors for delirium. Currently, there is no study reporting the prevalence of delirium after HSCT, but in adults, it is around 50% [34].

The treatment of delirium in this context is not specific and is based on non-pharmacological and risk factor reduction measures. In case of failure, atypical neuroleptics are recommended [10].

> Supportive treatment, and early detection and treatment of complications are important influencers of the outcome in patients with sinusoidal obstructive syndrome.

Other Causes of Liver Injury in Children Undergoing HSCT

The liver may suffer from multiple sequential or concurrent injuries, each comprising its own aetiology. With the broad spectrum of possible post-HSCT complications in mind, the clinician in the PICU will properly rank the priorities among the different organ toxicities. Notably, it is common after HSCT that treatment of one organ toxicity may increase the burden of toxicity on another suffering organ. It is especially true for the liver, which is a physiologic hub involved in many regulations.

Another very important aspect of HSCT is the sort of donor used. Autologous transplantation is usually a less complex setting compared to allogeneic HSCT in children. Notably, children transplanted with autologous HSCT are not at risk of acute or chronic GVHD, they do not suffer from kidney toxicities related to immunosuppressive drugs, since their immunodepression is less important and only lasts for 3 to 6 months after HSCT, and they are exceptionally at risk of viral hepatitis mediated by viral reactivation.

Also, medical management of post-HSCT children in PICU is based on the principle that time is a key element of a favourable outcome. Even for children with multiorgan failure and complex and intricated toxicities, buying time through aggressive management may allow the patient to reach the next milestone that will dramatically change his evolution: neutrophil recovery will control infections, antibiotics and antifungal discontinuation will help the liver and kidney to recover from toxicities, immunosuppressive medication will finally control severe acute GVHD.

Infection

Hepatotropic Virus

HSCT patients are at risk of acute hepatitis related to reactivation or primary viral infections of mainly CMV, less frequently adenovirus, EBV and very rarely HHV 6, HHV 7, VZV and herpes simplex virus (HSV). For patient with chronic hepatitis B or C viral infections before HSCT, there is also a risk of seroconversion associated hyperacute hepatitis at the time of immune recovery. The period and intensity of immunodepression depends on the conditioning regimen, the type of graft, the use of T-cell depletion graft and the occurrence of graft versus host disease (GVHD). It includes the period before engraftment as well as the 6 months that constitute the delay for immune reconstitution. Viral replication in the blood is generally detected from day 21 post HSCT. These viruses are responsible for liver damage ranging from discrete transaminase elevation to fulminant hepatitis [35].

Sepsis

There are two types of clinical pictures of liver damage in sepsis: hypoxic-ischemic hepatitis, a consequence of insufficient blood supply to the liver, and cholestatic liver dysfunction with accumulation of bilirubin and bile acids in the liver [36].

While clinical signs of sepsis are fairly obvious when there is low liver flow, cholestasis can be a frustrating symptom of sepsis and should always alarm about this possible diagnosis, especially in the context of post-HSCT.

Graft Versus Host Disease

Acute Graft Versus Host Disease

Acute graft-versus-host disease (aGVHD) occurs in 35–50% of patients after donor engraftment, typically within 100 days post HSCT. Donor's activated T-cells migrate to the main target tissues, which are the skin, gastrointestinal tract and liver. Liver damage is thus usually not isolated but it is concomitant of skin rash and digestive symptoms such as abdominal pain and diarrhoea [37]. Liver damage is characterized by cytolysis or cholestasis. There are four grades that determine aGVHD severity, depending on the stage by organ. Liver is staged on the degree of increase in bilirubin, an increase in bilirubin is at least grade II (Table 4).

Chronic Graft Versus Host Disease

Chronic graft versus host disease (cGVHD) affects 20–50% of patients, according to the definition, after 100 days post HSCT. The cellular mechanism is not perfectly identified but it involves alloreactive donor T-cells and B-cells. Median onset is about 6 months and cGVHD involves almost any organ of the body, but contrary to aGVHD, liver injury can be isolated. When this is the case, diagnosis can be difficult and requires ruling out all other potential causes of liver damage and may require a liver biopsy [38]. There are two forms of liver damage: the most frequent is characterized by a progressive cholestasis with severe lesions of the bile ducts

Table 4 Staging and grading of acute chronic graft versus host disease

Stage	Skin	Liver (bilirubin)	Gut (stool output/day)
0	No rash	<2 mg/dL	<10 mL//kg/day
1	Maculopapular rash <25% BSA	2–3 mg/dL	10–19.9 mL/kg/day
2	Maculopapular rash 25–50% BSA	3.1–6 mg/dL	20–30 mL/kg/day
3	Maculopapular rash >50% BSA	6.1–15 mg/dL	>30 mL/kg/day
4	Generalized erythroderma plus bullous formation	>15 mg/dL	Severe abdominal pain with or without ileus
Grade			
I	Stage 1–2	None	None
II	Stage 3, or	Stage 1, or	Stage 1
III	–	Stage 2–3, or	Stage 2–4
IV	Stage 4, or	Stage 4	–

BSA body surface area

leading to their destruction and constituting the "vanishing bile duct syndrome". The second, much rarer form, called "hepatitis GVHD", is characterized by an abrupt rise in transaminases, with, on biopsy, marked lobular hepatitis, sinusoidal inflammation and apoptosis of the hepatocytes [39].

Metabolic

Parenteral Nutrition-Associated Cholestasis

A hypercatabolic state related to chemotherapy, total body irradiation and GVHD as well as limited oral intake in the peri-HSCT period places the child at high risk of malnutrition. Enteral nutrition is recommended in first intention [23] but some patients will necessitate parenteral nutrition (PN). Even for short durations, parenteral nutrition is a cause of cholestasis, with a reported incidence of 15.7% in patients receiving PN for 14 to 30 days [40].

Iron Overload

Iron overload is rather responsible for long-term liver damage. The mechanisms involved are related to repeated pre-HSCT RBC transfusions in patients with transfusions-dependent anaemia, mobilization of iron from the bone marrow caused by regimen conditioning and repeated transfusions during the post-transplant aplasia period [41]. Free iron, by generating free radicals, leads to a pro-oxidant and pro-inflammatory state. Iron overload is associated with the acute phase with an increased rate of fungal and bacterial infections, an increased rate of acute GVHD and possibly an increased risk of SOS [42].

Drug-Related Injury

During the HSCT process, patients are likely to receive a number of hepatotoxic drugs. Given all the causes of liver impairment listed above, the responsibility for the drugs should be discussed, but all other causes should be investigated simultaneously. Key arguments necessary for the diagnosis of drug-related injury reported by Navarro et al. include: time to onset after initiation of treatment, elimination of another cause of liver injury, improvement in liver function after drug discontinuation and worsening on re-introduction [43]. Specific data concerning the toxicity of each drug is reported on the "LiverTox" website, produced by the National Institute of Diabetes and Digestive and Kidney Diseases [44].

Here we will focus on the anti-infectious therapeutics to which patients in post-HSCT are inevitably exposed.

Fungal prophylaxis is recommended for any patient undergoing HSCT during the granulocytopenic phase until engraftment and might be continued until immune recovery [45]. The various recommended options include first-generation triazoles (fluconazole and itraconazole), second-generation triazoles (voriconazole), echinocandins (mycafungin) and the liposomal form of amphotericin B. While most triazoles are associated with both cholestatic and cytolytic liver injury with voriconazole exposure-dependent hepatotoxicity, echinocandins and amphotericin B appear to be well tolerated [46].

As for the *antibiotics*, betalactamins are associated with hepatic alteration: penicillins are associated with acute hepatitis and with cholestasis, cephalosporins, ticarcillin and piperacillin are associated with a moderate increase in liver enzymes. It should be noted that ceftriaxone has a purely biliary elimination and may be responsible for biliary sludge and pseudolithiasis [47].

Altogether, these causes of liver injury (summarized above) can complicate the management of patients with sinusoidal obstructive syndrome.

Conclusions

Sinusoidal obstructive syndrome is common after marrow transplantation in children and requires admission to PICU in moderate forms progressing rapidly and severe forms. Its management is based on defibrotide and supportive care, especially aggressive fluid balance control. Besides, during HSCT, the liver is the target of multiple hits, which are metabolic, infectious and toxic. However, isolated complications observed in HSCT out of the association with SOS are rarely a cause for admission to the intensive care unit.

References

1. Zinter MS, Logan BR, Fretham C, Sapru A, Abraham A, Aljurf MD, et al. Comprehensive prognostication in critically ill pediatric hematopoietic cell transplant patients: results from merging the center for International Blood and Marrow Transplant Research (CIBMTR) and virtual Pediatric systems (VPS) registries. Biol Blood Marrow Transplant. 2020;26(2):333–42.
2. Gooley TA, Chien JW, Pergam SA, Hingorani S, Sorror ML, Boeckh M, et al. Reduced mortality after allogeneic hematopoietic-cell transplantation. N Engl J Med. 2010;363(22):2091–101.
3. Bratton SL, Van Duker H, Statler KD, Pulsipher MA, McArthur J, Keenan HT. Lower hospital mortality and complications after pediatric hematopoietic stem cell transplantation. Crit Care Med. 2008;36(3):923–7.
4. Chima RS, Daniels RC, Kim M-O, Li D, Wheeler DS, Davies SM, et al. Improved outcomes for stem cell transplant recipients requiring pediatric intensive care. Pediatr Crit Care Med. 2012;13(6):e336–42.

5. Lee SH, Yoo KH, Sung KW, Koo HH, Kwon YJ, Kwon MM, et al. Hepatic veno-occlusive disease in children after hematopoietic stem cell transplantation: incidence, risk factors, and outcome. Bone Marrow Transplant. 2010;45(8):1287–93.
6. Corbacioglu S, Carreras E, Ansari M, Balduzzi A, Cesaro S, Dalle J-H, et al. Diagnosis and severity criteria for sinusoidal obstruction syndrome/veno-occlusive disease in pediatric patients: a new classification from the European society for blood and marrow transplantation. Bone Marrow Transplant. 2018;53(2):138–45.
7. Mahadeo KM, Bajwa R, Abdel-Azim H, Lehmann LE, Duncan C, Zantek N, et al. Diagnosis, grading, and treatment recommendations for children, adolescents, and young adults with sinusoidal obstructive syndrome: an international expert position statement. Lancet Haematol. 2020;7(1):61–72. Available from: https://linkinghub.elsevier.com/retrieve/pii/S2352302619302017.
8. RPS B, Mahadeo KM, Taragin BH, Dvorak CC, McArthur J, Jeyapalan A, et al. Consensus report by Pediatric Acute Lung Injury and Sepsis Investigators and Pediatric Blood and Marrow Transplantation Consortium Joint Working Committees: supportive care guidelines for management of veno-occlusive disease in children and adolescents, part 1: focus on investigations, prophylaxis, and specific treatment. Biol Blood Marrow Transplant. 2017;23(11):1817–25. Available from: https://linkinghub.elsevier.com/retrieve/pii/S1083879117306122.
9. Mahadeo KM, McArthur J, Adams RH, Radhi M, Angelo J, Jeyapalan A, et al. Consensus report by the Pediatric Acute Lung Injury and Sepsis Investigators and Pediatric Blood and Marrow Transplant Consortium Joint Working Committees on supportive care guidelines for management of veno-occlusive disease in children and adolescents: part 2—focus on ascites, fluid and electrolytes, renal, and transfusion issues. Biol Blood Marrow Transplant. 2017;23(12):2023–33. Available from: https://linkinghub.elsevier.com/retrieve/pii/S1083879117306493.
10. Ovchinsky N, Frazier W, Auletta JJ, Dvorak CC, Ardura M, Song E, et al. Consensus report by the Pediatric Acute Lung Injury and Sepsis Investigators and Pediatric Blood and Marrow Transplantation Consortium Joint Working Committees on supportive care guidelines for management of veno-occlusive disease in children and adolescents, part 3: focus on cardiorespiratory dysfunction, infections, liver dysfunction, and delirium. Biol Blood Marrow Transplant. 2018;24(2):207–18. Available from: https://linkinghub.elsevier.com/retrieve/pii/S1083879117306900.
11. Corbacioglu S, Greil J, Peters C, Wulffraat N, Laws HJ, Dilloo D, et al. Defibrotide in the treatment of children with veno-occlusive disease (VOD): a retrospective multicentre study demonstrates therapeutic efficacy upon early intervention. Bone Marrow Transplant. 2004;33(2):189–95.
12. Faraci M, Bertaina A, Luksch R, Calore E, Lanino E, Saglio F, et al. Sinusoidal obstruction syndrome/Veno-occlusive disease after autologous or allogeneic hematopoietic stem cell transplantation in children: a retrospective study of the Italian Hematology-oncology association-hematopoietic stem cell transplantation group. Biol Blood Marrow Transplant. 2019;25(2):313–20.
13. Seifert C, Wittig S, Arndt C, Gruhn B. Heparanase polymorphisms: influence on incidence of hepatic sinusoidal obstruction syndrome in children undergoing allogeneic hematopoietic stem cell transplantation. J Cancer Res Clin Oncol. 2015;141(5):877–85. Available from: http://link.springer.com/10.1007/s00432-014-1857-2.
14. on behalf of the Paediatric Disease Working Parties of the European Blood and Marrow Transplant group, Huezo-Diaz Curtis P, Uppugunduri CRS, Muthukumaran J, Rezgui MA, Peters C, et al. Association of CTH variant with sinusoidal obstruction syndrome in children receiving intravenous busulfan and cyclophosphamide before hematopoietic stem cell transplantation. Pharmacogenomics J. 2018;18(1):64–9. Available from: http://www.nature.com/articles/tpj201665.
15. Corbacioglu S, Jabbour EJ, Mohty M. Risk factors for development of and progression of hepatic veno-occlusive disease/sinusoidal obstruction syndrome. Biol Blood Marrow

Transplant. 2019;25(7):1271–80. Available from: https://linkinghub.elsevier.com/retrieve/pii/S1083879119301430.
16. McKoy JM, Angelotta C, Bennett CL, Tallman MS, Wadleigh M, Evens AM, et al. Gemtuzumab ozogamicin-associated sinusoidal obstructive syndrome (SOS): an overview from the research on adverse drug events and reports (RADAR) project. Leuk Res. 2007;31(5):599–604.
17. Wadleigh M, Richardson PG, Zahrieh D, Lee SJ, Cutler C, Ho V, et al. Prior gemtuzumab ozogamicin exposure significantly increases the risk of veno-occlusive disease in patients who undergo myeloablative allogeneic stem cell transplantation. Blood. 2003;102(5):1578–82.
18. Kebriaei P, Wilhelm K, Ravandi F, Brandt M, de Lima M, Ciurea S, et al. Feasibility of allografting in patients with advanced acute lymphoblastic leukemia after salvage therapy with inotuzumab ozogamicin. Clin Lymphoma Myeloma Leuk. 2013;13(3):296–301.
19. Corbacioglu S, Hönig M, Lahr G, Stöhr S, Berry G, Friedrich W, et al. Stem cell transplantation in children with infantile osteopetrosis is associated with a high incidence of VOD, which could be prevented with defibrotide. Bone Marrow Transplant. 2006;38(8):547–53. Available from: http://www.nature.com/articles/1705485.
20. Naples JC, Skeens MA, Auletta J, Rangarajan H, Abu-Arja R, Horwitz E, et al. Anicteric veno-occlusive disease after hematopoietic stem cell transplantation in children. Bone Marrow Transplant. 2016;51(1):135–7.
21. Benoit G, Phan V, Duval M, Champagne M, Litalien C, Merouani A. Fluid balance of pediatric hematopoietic stem cell transplant recipients and intensive care unit admission. Pediatr Nephrol. 2007;22(3):441–7.
22. Rondón G, Saliba RM, Chen J, Ledesma C, Alousi AM, Oran B, et al. Impact of fluid overload as new toxicity category on hematopoietic stem cell transplantation outcomes. Biol Blood Marrow Transplant. 2017;23(12):2166–71.
23. Nava T, Ansari M, Dalle J-H, de Heredia CD, Güngör T, Trigoso E, et al. Supportive care during pediatric hematopoietic stem cell transplantation: beyond infectious diseases. A report from workshops on supportive care of the Pediatric Diseases Working Party (PDWP) of the European Society for Blood and Marrow Transplantation (EBMT). Bone Marrow Transplant. 2020;55(6):1126–36. Available from: http://www.nature.com/articles/s41409-020-0818-4.
24. Duncan C, Kahn J, Grupp SA, Richardson PG. Recent developments with defibrotide for the treatment of hepatic veno-occlusive disease/sinusoidal obstruction syndrome. Expert Opin Orphan Drugs. 2019;7(7–8):337–47. Available from: https://www.tandfonline.com/doi/full/10.1080/21678707.2019.1651641.
25. Valentine SL, Bembea MM, Muszynski JA, Cholette JM, Doctor A, Spinella PC, et al. Consensus recommendations for RBC transfusion practice in critically ill children from the pediatric critical care transfusion and anemia expertise initiative. Pediatr Crit Care Med. 2018;19(9):884–98.
26. Robitaille N, Lacroix J, Alexandrov L, Clayton L, Cortier M, Schultz KR, et al. Excess of veno-occlusive disease in a randomized clinical trial on a higher trigger for red blood cell transfusion after bone marrow transplantation: a Canadian blood and marrow transplant group trial. Biol Blood Marrow Transplant. 2013;19(3):468–73. Available from: https://linkinghub.elsevier.com/retrieve/pii/S108387911201138X.
27. Pediatric Acute Lung Injury Consensus Conference Group. Pediatric acute respiratory distress syndrome: consensus recommendations from the Pediatric acute lung injury consensus conference. Pediatr Crit Care Med. 2015;16(5):428–39.
28. Gow KW, Wulkan ML, Heiss KF, Haight AE, Heard ML, Rycus P, et al. Extracorporeal membrane oxygenation for support of children after hematopoietic stem cell transplantation: the Extracorporeal Life Support Organization experience. J Pediatr Surg. 2006;41(4):662–7. Available from: https://linkinghub.elsevier.com/retrieve/pii/S0022346805009486.
29. Di Nardo M, Locatelli F, Palmer K, Amodeo A, Lorusso R, Belliato M, et al. Extracorporeal membrane oxygenation in pediatric recipients of hematopoietic stem cell transplantation: an updated analysis of the extracorporeal life support organization experience. Intensive Care Med. 2014;40(5):754–6.

30. Strouse C, Richardson P, Prentice G, Korman S, Hume R, Nejadnik B, et al. Defibrotide for treatment of severe veno-occlusive disease in pediatrics and adults: an exploratory analysis using data from the Center for International Blood and Marrow Transplant Research. Biol Blood Marrow Transplant. 2016;22(7):1306–12. Available from: https://linkinghub.elsevier.com/retrieve/pii/S1083879116300301.
31. Raanani P, Gafter-Gvili A, Paul M, Ben-Bassat I, Leibovici L, Shpilberg O. Immunoglobulin prophylaxis in hematopoietic stem cell transplantation: systematic review and meta-analysis. J Clin Oncol. 2009;27(5):770–81. Available from: http://ascopubs.org/doi/10.1200/JCO.2008.16.8450.
32. Nimer SD, Milewicz AL, Champlin RE, Busuttil RW. Successful treatment of hepatic veno-occlusive disease in a bone marrow transplant patient with orthotopic liver transplantation. Transplantation. 1990;49(4):819–21.
33. Mellgren K, Fasth A, Saalman R, Olausson M, Abrahamsson J. Liver transplantation after stem cell transplantation with the same living donor in a monozygotic twin with acute myeloid leukemia. Ann Hematol. 2005;84(11):755–7.
34. Fann JR, Roth-Roemer S, Burington BE, Katon WJ, Syrjala KL. Delirium in patients undergoing hematopoietic stem cell transplantation. Cancer. 2002;95(9):1971–81.
35. Locasciulli A, Nava S, Sparano P, Testa M. Infections with hepatotropic viruses in children treated with allogeneic bone marrow transplantation. Bone Marrow Transplant. 1998;21(Suppl 2):S75–7.
36. Jenniskens M, Langouche L, Vanwijngaerden Y-M, Mesotten D, Van den Berghe G. Cholestatic liver (dys)function during sepsis and other critical illnesses. Intensive Care Med. 2016;42(1):16–27.
37. Jacobsohn DA, Vogelsang GB. Acute graft versus host disease. Orphanet J Rare Dis. 2007;2:35.
38. Baird K, Cooke K, Schultz KR. Chronic graft-versus-host disease (GVHD) in children. Pediatr Clin N Am. 2010;57(1):297–322.
39. Melín-Aldana H, Thormann K, Duerst R, Kletzel M, Jacobsohn DA. Hepatitic pattern of graft versus host disease in children. Pediatr Blood Cancer. 2007;49(5):727–30.
40. Lauriti G, Zani A, Aufieri R, Cananzi M, Chiesa PL, Eaton S, et al. Incidence, prevention, and treatment of parenteral nutrition-associated cholestasis and intestinal failure-associated liver disease in infants and children: a systematic review. JPEN J Parenter Enteral Nutr. 2014;38(1):70–85.
41. Majhail NS, Lazarus HM, Burns LJ. Iron overload in hematopoietic cell transplantation. Bone Marrow Transplant. 2008;41(12):997–1003.
42. Jastaniah W, Harmatz P, Pakbaz Z, Fischer R, Vichinsky E, Walters MC. Transfusional iron burden and liver toxicity after bone marrow transplantation for acute myelogenous leukemia and hemoglobinopathies. Pediatr Blood Cancer. 2008;50(2):319–24.
43. Navarro VJ, Senior JR. Drug-related hepatotoxicity. N Engl J Med. 2006;354(7):731–9.
44. National Institute of Diabetes and Digestive and Kidney Diseases. LiverTox [Internet]. Available from: livertox.nih.gov.
45. Groll AH, Castagnola E, Cesaro S, Dalle J-H, Engelhard D, Hope W, et al. Fourth European Conference on Infections in Leukaemia (ECIL-4): guidelines for diagnosis, prevention, and treatment of invasive fungal diseases in paediatric patients with cancer or allogeneic haemopoietic stem-cell transplantation. Lancet Oncol. 2014;15(8):e327–40.
46. Kyriakidis I, Tragiannidis A, Munchen S, Groll AH. Clinical hepatotoxicity associated with antifungal agents. Expert Opin Drug Saf. 2017;16(2):149–65.
47. Lagacé-Wiens P, Rubinstein E. Adverse reactions to β-lactam antimicrobials. Expert Opin Drug Saf. 2012;11(3):381–99.

Liver Transplantation in Critically Ill Children

Massimiliano Paganelli

In children as in adults, liver transplantation (LT) is the standard of care for end-stage liver disease. Over the last 20 years, the advancement of surgical techniques, liver disease prioritization, and better immunosuppression regimens led to very successful outcomes for most children and adolescents undergoing the procedure. The improvement of pre- and posttransplant intensive care played a crucial role in increasing the overall survival and reducing morbidity, especially for patients suffering from acute or acute-on-chronic liver failure. In this chapter we address the main aspects to consider when caring for infants, children, and adolescents before and after LT.

Main Aspects of Liver Transplantation in Children

Surgical Approaches

Surgical approaches to pediatric LT have significantly evolved since Thomas Starzl's first case in 1963 [1]. Transplantation of size-matched whole livers, which was limited by the scarcity of appropriate-sized organs, was gradually replaced by reduced-size grafts, which allows even small children to receive LT from adult donors. Whole liver transplantation (WLT) went from being almost 100% of pediatric LT in the 1980s to representing <60% of procedures in North America and <30% of LT in Europe in the last 10 years [2–4]. Transplantation of left lateral

M. Paganelli (✉)
Pediatric Hepatology, CHU Sainte-Justine, Université de Montréal, Montreal, QC, Canada

Liver Tissue Engineering and Cell Therapy Laboratory, CHU Sainte-Justine Research Center, Montreal, QC, Canada
e-mail: m.paganelli@umontreal.ca

P. Jouvet, F. Alvarez (eds.), *Liver Diseases in the Pediatric Intensive Care Unit*,
https://doi.org/10.1007/978-3-030-79132-2_10

segmental grafts (LLS, Couinaud's segments 2 and 3) is now the most common type of LT for small children, WLT being mostly reserved for older children and adolescents. LLS are traditionally obtained by reducing adult donors' organs. Nevertheless, this approach results in using only part of the organ, wasting the entirety of the right lobe. Since small children represent the biggest proportion of pediatric LT receivers, such a strategy negatively impacts adult patients on the waiting list. Significant progress to tackle the problem of organ shortage was achieved with the diffusion of split LT (SLT), consisting in the division of the deceased donor liver into two transplantable grafts, and living donor LT (LDLT). The latter results from the transplant of children with LLS resected from healthy adult donors. Combination of SLT and LDLT now represents almost 70% of pediatric LT in Europe, 40% in North America, and >95% in Japan [2, 4, 5]. LDLT was developed to answer cadaveric organ shortage. First accomplished in 1988, LDLT provides significant advantages on WLT (reduction of ischemia) and on SLT (most notably shorter wait time and preoperative control of graft steatosis through diet and exercise) [6, 7]. The experience of LDLT led to the extension of the in situ division of the liver parenchyma technique to SLT and LLS procurement. This approach shortens the ischemia time (essential when organs are shared across very large territories) and improves the control of bleeding, at the expense of an increased surgical complexity and operation time [8]. Anyhow, the surgical approach depends also on recipient- and donor-related anatomic issues. Special conditions such as portal vein thrombosis or tumor extension in the recipient, or vascular anomalies in the donor, impact the surgical strategy. In some selected centers, partial orthotopic liver transplantation, which consists in replacing a portion of the native liver by a size-matched partial graft, leaving the rest of the recipient's liver in place, has provided interesting results for children with acute liver failure (ALF), and is a still controverted option for some inborn errors of liver metabolism [9]. By temporarily restoring liver functions, partial LT represents a bridge to native liver regeneration for selected patients with ALF, ready to be explanted as soon as the patient's own liver recovers, avoiding lifelong immunosuppression.

> The choice of the surgical approach to LT depends on the recipient's underlying diagnosis and clinical condition, the donor characteristics, local surgical expertise, and organ allocation policies

Donor Selection

When selecting donors for pediatric LT, several factors need to be considered. First of all the size of the graft needs to provide sufficient parenchymal mass to restore the function while avoiding the complications related to the transplantation of an organ too big to accommodate a child's abdominal cavity. The minimal hepatic mass needed has not been clearly established and depends on the standard liver volume of the recipient and the size of the donor's organ and of its LLS. Since preservation injury is more important in deceased donors, the calculated mass necessary for reduced-size or split liver grafts is usually greater than the mass needed for LDLT. A small-for-size graft syndrome develops when the graft volume is insufficient for the recipient's metabolic demands. To avoid this, a graft-to-recipient weight ratio ≥0.8% (ideally 1–4%) or a donor-to-recipient standard liver volume ratio ≥40% are recommended [10, 11]. Whereas calculation of the former requires the actual weight of the graft, which complicates organ allocation, estimation of the latter is only based on body surface area (standard liver volume = 706.2 x body surface area + 2.4) [11]. In daily practice, many centers rely on donor-to-recipient weight ratio (DRWR) to quickly assess the suitability of potential donors. Although no clear guidelines exist, donors are considered suitable for pediatric WLT if the resulting DRWR is between 0.5 and 2. Since LLS accounts for 25–30% of the total liver volume, the accepted DRWR for SLT and LDLT is usually between 2 and 12 [2]. Interestingly, a recent analysis of the liver transplant wait-list in the U.S. revealed that 50% of the organs that were declined for size resulted to be in the ideal range for size match by body surface area [12]. Hyper-reduced grafts and monosegmental grafts open the possibility to transplant very small infants using cadaveric or living adult donors without the complications of large-for-size grafts. Nevertheless, such approaches require advanced surgical skills that are not developed in all transplant centers.

Liver donor–recipient matching is based on ABO compatibility. Nevertheless, although associated with a greater rate of complications, the use of ABO-incompatible donors is sometimes considered for young children (<1.5–2 years) in critical conditions, with identical outcome in terms of graft survival [13]. Pretreatment with rituximab and plasmapheresis exchange and a more aggressive immunosuppressive regimen led to significant improvements in graft survival after LDLT even for older children [7].

Donor organ quality has a significant impact on the success of LT. Donors should be young (older than 3–6 months of age and ideally <40 years if LDLT or SLT are considered) and not obese, with near-normal liver function tests (≤2–3 times the upper limit of the normal), have no history of liver disease, an intensive care unit stay <5 days and be hemodynamically stable [14]. Whereas the use of livers from older donors does not seem to be associated with worse short-term outcome in adult recipients, a higher incidence of intrahepatic biliary strictures has been described for pediatric recipients [15, 16]. Although livers with >20% macrovesicular steatosis are associated with an increased risk of allograft loss, the use of organs from overweight and obese donors (BMI 25–35 kg/m^2), but not from severely obese donors (BMI >35), does not result in decreased graft or patient survival [17, 18]. The impact of donor's liver steatosis on postoperative outcome is greater in case of graft reduction (for which >10% macrovesicular steatosis at biopsy is usually considered a relative contraindication) or long cold ischemia time. Whereas the use of livers from donors with hypernatremia has been associated with an increased risk of graft dysfunction and poor outcome in adults, pediatric data showed no increase in mortality or complications and suggest that it might be acceptable [19, 20].

In the case of LDLT, donor well-being is the primary focus, and it is assured by delegating donor selection and evaluation to an independent team. A fully informed consent, absence of any coercion, and the possibility to opt out at any time are mainstays of the process. The criteria listed above are also applicable to living-related donor selection, with the added advantage of disposing of more time to test for genetic conditions in the case of LT for metabolic disorders. Nevertheless, accelerated living donor evaluation in <48 h can be safely achieved for children with ALF in those centers with a carefully organized process in place.

Overall, although decision support models have been and are being designed, no clear rule exists and each cadaveric donor must be assessed by balancing the quality of the organ with the health status of the potential recipient [21–23]. The consequences of accepting high-risk organs on posttransplant morbidity and mortality should be properly weighted, always taking into consideration the long life expectancy of children undergoing LT. Nevertheless, it is important to remember that 55% of the children that died on the liver transplant wait-list in the U.S. had been offered an organ that was refused and eventually transplanted into another pediatric recipient [12].

Outcomes and Surgical Complications

More than 50 years after the first operation was performed in a child, pediatric LT has become a very successful procedure that has transformed the prognosis of children with end-stage liver disease. Current 1-year survival rate after LT is >95% for chronic conditions and >85% for ALF in most reference centers worldwide (Fig. 1).

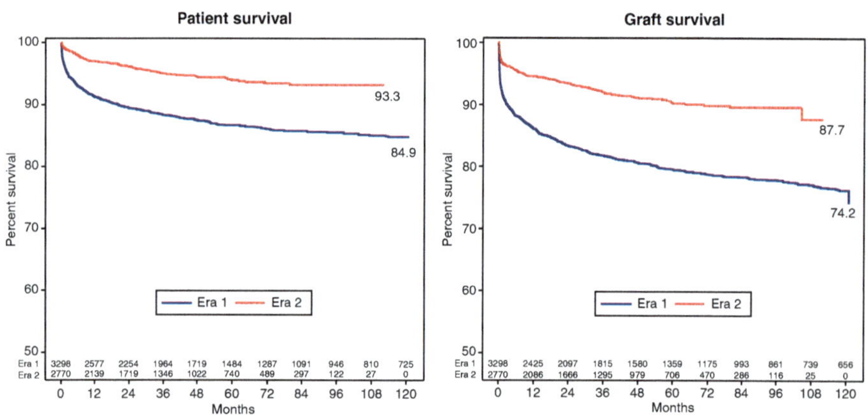

Fig. 1 Kaplan-Meier plot of patient (left) and graft (right) survival after pediatric liver transplantation by era (data from the Society of Pediatric Liver Transplantation). Era 1 includes all the patients who received their first transplant between Jan 1995 and Dec 2009, and Era 2 is defined as any transplant after Jan 2011. The number of participants at risk of event over time is reported above the x axis (data lock 21 September 2020) [3]

Long-term patient and graft survival progressively improved with the introduction of more effective immunosuppressive regimens and refinement of surgical techniques and donor selection criteria. Recently published large series describes 20-year patient and graft survival rates of 69–79% and 53–64%, respectively, with better results observed for nonurgent indications and up to 80% graft survival in children undergoing LDLT for biliary atresia [24–26]. Reported outcomes are overall similar between WLT and reduced-liver variants, with LDLT being comparable to WLT for both short and long-term graft and patient survival [4, 27, 28]. Nevertheless, incidence of vascular thrombosis and retransplantation were reported to be lower in small recipient receiving technical variant allografts (especially LDLT) compared to WLT, with better 1-, 5-, and 10-year graft survival [29]. Graft survival 5 years after pediatric LT is now >80% (about 80% for ALF and >87% for biliary atresia, and closer to 90% after LDLT in most experienced centers), and >65% after retransplantation [28, 30].

Upon reperfusion of the graft, liver function progressively recovers, leading to a rapid improvement of the patient's conditions. In rare occasions (up to 7% of pediatric LT), the graft fails soon after reperfusion, without an identifiable cause. What is defined as primary nonfunction rapidly leads to death if no urgent retransplantation is performed. Long warm ischemia time, patient's hemodynamic instability, and low cardiac output have been identified as risk factors. Theoretical spontaneous recovery of the graft is possible, as in ALF, if the patient survives long enough to allow for the organ's regeneration. When graft dysfunction is milder and progressively resolves without the need for retransplantation, it is defined as early graft dysfunction.

Surgical complications after LT are common, require prompt multidisciplinary management and can occasionally lead to graft loss and even patient death. Biliary complications, such as biliary leaks, anastomotic, and non-anastomotic strictures or excluded bile ducts, represent the most frequent surgical problem after pediatric LT, overall affecting 10–30% of the recipients (Table 1) [31]. Incidence of such complications is traditionally reported to be higher for reduced-size grafts, although differences are minimized by surgical experience [31–33]. Since bile ducts are perfused only by the hepatic arterial flow, ischemia is the main risk factor for biliary complications. Liver parenchymal reduction put the vascularization of the left hepatic duct at risk. Moreover, bile ducts are more susceptible to ischemia damage because of the presence of bile salts in its lumen that attack the biliary epithelium. This is amplified by any arterial complication, such as thrombosis or stenosis. While biliary leaks usually manifest in the first week after LT with clear signs, stenoses present later, with absent or mild symptoms and sometimes very subtle signs (with >50% of the patients not showing bile duct dilation) [34]. Treatment of biliary complications needs to be aggressive in order to avoid secondary biliary cirrhosis and graft loss. Whereas surgical approach is usually preferred for biliary leaks, a less-invasive radiological interventional approach with long-term, temporary stenting can provide excellent results for biliary stenoses in experienced centers [32, 34].

Biliary leaks and strictures represent a frequent complication, increasing post-transplant morbidity

Table 1 Summary of vascular and biliary complications at 30 and 90 days

	Donor organ type				
	Live $N = 972$	Whole $N = 3263$	Reduced $N = 785$	Split $N = 873$	Total $N = 5893$
Total early follow-up assessment					
Total at 30 days	953	3167	761	847	5728
Total at 90 days	493	1556	273	462	2784
Portal vein thrombosis 30 days					
Yes	46 (4.8%)	92 (2.9%)	48 (6.3%)	46 (5.4%)	232 (4.1%)
No	717 (75.2%)	2350 (74.2%)	548 (72.0%)	670 (79.1%)	4285 (74.8%)
Missing	190 (19.9%)	725 (22.9%)	165 (21.7%)	131 (15.5%)	1211 (21.1%)
Portal vein thrombosis 30–90 days					
Yes	3 (0.6%)	1 (0.1%)	0	1 (0.2%)	5 (0.2%)
No	332 (67.3%)	998 (64.1%)	134 (49.1%)	300 (64.9%)	1764 (63.4%)
Missing	44 (8.9%)	171 (11.0%)	57 (20.9%)	35 (7.6%)	307 (11.0%)
Data not collected	114 (23.1%)	386 (24.8%)	82 (30.0%)	126 (27.3%)	708 (25.4%)
Hepatic artery thrombosis 30 days					
Yes	49 (5.1%)	259 (8.2%)	48 (6.3%)	40 (4.7%)	396 (6.9%)
No	711 (74.6%)	2185 (69.0%)	548 (72.0%)	676 (79.8%)	4120 (71.9%)
Missing	193 (20.3%)	723 (22.8%)	165 (21.7%)	131 (15.5%)	1212 (21.2%)
Hepatic artery thrombosis 30–90 days					
Yes	2 (0.4%)	6 (0.4%)	0	1 (0.2%)	9 (0.3%)
No	333 (67.5%)	993 (63.8%)	134 (49.1%)	300 (64.9%)	1760 (63.2%)
Missing	44 (8.9%)	171 (11.0%)	57 (20.9%)	35 (7.6%)	307 (11.0%)
Data not collected	114 (23.1%)	386 (24.8%)	82 (30.0%)	126 (27.3%)	708 (25.4%)
Biliary complications 30 days					
Yes	140 (14.7%)	269 (8.5%)	119 (15.6%)	147 (17.4%)	675 (11.8%)
No	496 (52.0%)	1756 (55.4%)	397 (52.2%)	436 (51.5%)	3085 (53.9%)
Missing	188 (19.7%)	709 (22.4%)	165 (21.7%)	129 (15.2%)	1191 (20.8%)
Data not collected	129 (13.5%)	433 (13.7%)	80 (10.5%)	135 (15.9%)	777 (13.6%)
Biliary complications 30–90 days					
Yes	29 (5.9%)	45 (2.9%)	24 (8.8%)	35 (7.6%)	133 (4.8%)
No	422 (85.6%)	1335 (85.8%)	189 (69.2%)	392 (84.8%)	2338 (84.0%)
Missing	42 (8.5%)	176 (11.3%)	60 (22.0%)	35 (7.6%)	313 (11.2%)

Data from the Society of Pediatric Liver Transplantation
Data where donor organ type is missing is excluded from these analyses *(data lock 21 September 2020)* [3]

Vascular complications are not rare and a source of significant morbidity (Table 1). Hepatic artery thrombosis (HAT) develops in 5–8% of patients and is the main cause of graft loss after pediatric LT [31, 35]. Similar incidence was observed for WLT, SLT, or LDLT [31, 36]. Although prolonged ischemia, cytomegalovirus infection, or hypercoagulable state are known risk factors for early HAT, technical issues (kinking, narrow anastomosis, small arteries, or mismatched vessel size), as well as a graft-to-recipient weight ratio >4%, are the most commonly identified cause [37]. Early HAT presents in the first 10 days after LT, usually with bile duct necrosis and subsequent necrosis of the liver and sepsis. Urgent retransplantation is required to save the patient's life. Nevertheless, especially in children, HAT can present in a more subtle way, with delayed biliary leak or intermittent septic episodes related to bile duct injury.

Preventing screening for HAT by Doppler ultrasonography during the first week post-LT allows for an early detection of HAT and aggressive treatment. Considering the high mortality, retransplantation is the treatment of choice, but revascularization, either surgical or endovascular, is usually attempted to gain time [38]. Portal vein complications, of which portal vein thrombosis (PVT) is the most severe, affect 3–8% of patients after pediatric LT [31, 39]. Reduced-size grafts, a graft-to-recipient weight ratio >4%, as well size discrepancies between donor and recipient and the use of cryopreserved interposition vascular grafts are associated with an increased incidence of PVT [31, 40, 41]. A small portal vein in the recipient, usually found in patients with biliary atresia, and abundance of portosystemic shunts (which reduce blood flow through the portal vein) are significant risk factors for PVT [42, 43]. Early PVT presents as graft dysfunction, which can be mild or severe enough to result in acute graft failure and require urgent retransplantation. Late-onset PVT is usually silent, with progressive portal hypertension developing with all its complications. Anticoagulation is usually tried but it is rarely effective, and surgical thrombectomy and reconstruction of the portal anastomosis is the treatment of choice. Interventional radiological approach is usually preferred for late-onset PVT, but it is increasingly being considered for early PVT as well. Unlike HAT and PVT, complete hepatic vein outflow obstruction (presenting as an acute Budd-Chiari syndrome) is a very rare complication. Nevertheless, incomplete obstruction resulting in prolonged ascites (which is an otherwise common and spontaneously resolving phenomenon after pediatric LT) is more often diagnosed at Doppler ultrasonography (especially with reduced-size grafts) and treated by endovascular dilation [39, 44].

Waiting for a Transplant

End-stage liver disease resulting from different acute or chronic conditions is the main indication for LT. Once the need for LT is identified, the patient is evaluated to assess his/her eligibility, identify causes for potential complications, put in place preventive measures to optimize the outcome and minimize wait-list mortality. Although most of the patients can afford to wait for LT at home, pretransplant decompensations requiring intensive care are not rare, while some children with most severe or acute conditions require close monitoring in the pediatric intensive care unit (PICU).

Indications

Chronic cholestatic diseases constitute the most frequent indication for pediatric liver transplantation, with biliary atresia alone justifying 33–40% of transplants in North America [3, 30]. Progression towards liver failure following chronic viral or autoimmune hepatitis accounts for only 3% of transplants, while inborn errors of liver metabolism and liver tumors are responsible for 14% and 8% of them, respectively. About 6–13% of liver transplants are performed for ALF, whereas acute decompensation of chronic conditions due to infectious complications or gastrointestinal bleeding (acute-on-chronic liver failure, ACLF) are less frequent in children, although also less well identified in available registries.

Pretransplant Evaluation and Listing

Pretransplant evaluation is a standardized process that allows the multidisciplinary transplant team to thoroughly assess the patient's physical and psychological condition, and sometimes reassess the underlying diagnosis [45]. Conducted with the participation of several pediatric subspecialists, the process examines every system to pinpoint potential contraindications, identify problems requiring immediate treatment and flag conditions that might increase the pre-, peri-, and postoperative risk of developing specific complications. The evaluation allows surgeons, hepatologists, and intensive care specialists to better know the patient and his/her family, and define the best strategy for LT. It also allows infectious disease specialists, cardiologists, hematologists, pulmonologists, nephrologists, endocrinologists, nutritionists, and dentists to put in place and carry out preventive measures and procedures (e.g.. vaccination) to avoid or limit complications. Other specialists, such as oncologists, neurologists, geneticists, or experts in metabolic diseases are involved for specific indications. Psychosocial assessment of patient and family is also crucial part of the process. The evaluation also allows the family and the patient to familiarize with the team, ask questions and fully understand (and prepare for) potential complications, and the risk of death. Visiting the facilities, and especially the PICU, is part of the process. The transplant coordinator plays a pivotal role in this process, assuring that all exams and consultations are successfully performed in a short period of time while limiting the stress on the family. The coordinator establishes him/herself as the main contact for the patient and family, designs with them the logistics of the pretransplant follow-up and actions upon an organ offer and, in case of LDLT, coordinate with the medical team evaluating the donor. The results of the evaluation are then gathered and presented to the review board in order to decide on the patient's listing for LT. Once the process is well established, in case of ALF or ACLF, the evaluation can be accelerated and conducted over a few hours to allow for an expedited listing.

Organ allocation is based on strictly regulated criteria that vary from country to country. For adults, it is most often based on the model for end-stage liver disease (MELD) score or its derivatives (e.g. MELD-Na), which objectively consider several clinical criteria (total bilirubin, international normalized ratio [INR], and creatinine) to establish the patient's risk of death at 3 months [46]. Pediatric liver disease prioritization is often based on MELD score (≥12 years of age) and on the pediatric end-stage liver disease (PELD) score for younger children. The latter adds growth failure, age <1 year, and albumin plasma levels to the equation, without creatinine [47, 48]. Some countries and provinces do not use MELD/PELD for pediatric patients and give priority to children on most adult recipients. Children with ACLF or very severe chronic conditions have priority on the list, although maximum priority is given to pediatric patients with ALF. Most countries have organ allocation policies allocating livers from pediatric donors to children first [49]. Exceptions scores are assigned for liver tumors, HAT, hepatopulmonary syndrome, and portopulmonary hypertension, and several genetic and metabolic diseases prioritize children that would otherwise suffer from severe morbidity. Other exceptions can be accepted after review from an independent board.

Pretransplant Management and Complications on the Waiting List

During the days or months separating the listing of a patient for transplant to the actual operation, the focus of caregivers is centered on preventing and managing complications. Portal hypertension, with ascites, hepatic encephalopathy (HE) and esophageal varices, poses the biggest risk and requires careful therapeutic follow-up with diuretics, laxatives, and nonabsorbable antibiotics, periodical albumin perfusion, and prophylactic endoscopic variceal banding to avoid potentially severe decompensations or bleeding. Occasional septic complications, often related to spontaneous bacterial peritonitis or cholangitis, are not unusual and might temporarily preclude LT, requiring temporary inactivation on the list. Pruritus, osteopenia, and impaired bone metabolism related to severe cholestasis need prompt treatment and supplementation to prevent pathologic fractures and improve the quality of life. Early diagnosis of HE and hepatorenal or, more rarely, hepatopulmonary syndrome or portopulmonary hypertension, is crucial to start adequate medical management and adapt prioritization on the waiting list. Although close pretransplant follow-up allows for outpatient management of many of these complications, patients often experience recurrent hospitalizations, and intensive care is often required during decompensations to treat septic shock or provide renal replacement therapy for hepatorenal syndrome or HE. The patient nutritional status needs special focus before LT. Growth failure and sarcopenia have an important impact on posttransplant outcome, especially for younger children, and are often underestimated by MELD/PELD score calculation [50, 51]. Thorough assessment, aggressive nutritional treatment, often requiring nasogastric tube feeding or parenteral nutrition, and, when possible, exercise are needed to optimize caloric intake and accelerate posttransplant recovery. Since sarcopenia increases the risk of developing HE and protein restriction has been demonstrated not to be necessary in patients with HE, protein intake should be optimized to the nutritional needs of the patient [51–53].

Nutritional status before the transplant is determinant in diminishing post-transplant morbidity and improving chances of survival

Post-transplant Management

Early management after pediatric LT requires close monitoring in the PICU. Whereas restoration of liver functions usually occurs over few hours after organ reperfusion, the complexity of extrahepatic organs involvement and the need for preventing and early identifying not-so-rare and potentially life-threatening complications make posttransplant monitoring resource-intensive.

Liver Function

Recovery of liver function starts soon after reperfusion of the organ and progresses rapidly. Serum aminotransferases remain high, or even increase, for a few days after LT (especially for segmental grafts), and, alone, should not be considered as sign of complications or underlying problems with graft recovery. Similarly, γ-glutamyltransferase (GGT) levels typically transiently increase after LT, and subsequently slowly decrease to normal levels over several days or weeks. Because of the slow clearance of delta-bilirubin, serum bilirubin levels take several weeks to decrease independently from graft functional recovery. Coagulation abnormalities are also common during the first 48 h from LT, although progressive improvement of the INR is expected, and no correction is usually required. Serum lactate and ammonia levels are considered reliable markers of graft function and should be monitored closely over the first 24–48 h. Neurological recovery is another important sign of improving graft function and, even when prolonged sedation is required for the management of extrahepatic complications, proper and recurrent assessment of sedation needs after LT is important.

Monitoring Potential Complications

Close monitoring in the PICU of all LT recipients for 24–48 h is required for an early detection of the potential complications listed above, which, when considered together, affect >50% of the patients [31]. Early postoperative hemorrhage is not uncommon after LT, with patients with portal hypertension and adhesions from previous abdominal surgeries being at higher risk. Abdominal drainage should be frequently measured, and the risk for surgical reassessment should be balanced against the evidence showing a negative impact of perioperative transfusions on survival [54]. Absence of clinical and biochemical improvement over the first hours from transplant should raise the suspicion of serious complications such as primary non-function, HAT or PVT (see above), which should be promptly excluded. Slow improvement over the first week after LT might hide vascular complications or an early graft dysfunction. Aggressive screening for vascular problems by Doppler ultrasonography (every 12 h, if possible, for the first 5 days and then daily for 5–7 days) is warranted to quickly identify complications. Vasopressors should be withdrawn as soon as possible to reduce the risk of thrombosis and, if no active bleeding detected, prophylaxis with heparin should be started within 24 h from LT, to be subsequently switched for acetylsalicylic acid once the risk of bleeding reduced.

Although ascites after pediatric LT is frequently observed after uncomplicated procedures, it might also be a sign of vascular and biliary complications. Periodical confirmation of its sterility and characterization of its composition by measuring bilirubin and triglyceride levels allow for early detection and subsequent treatment of bowel perforations, biliary leaks, and chylous ascites [44].

Careful screening and prophylaxis for potential infections is also a crucial part of the posttransplant management. Surgery, induction of immunosuppression, ascites, and the presence of invasive equipment make the patient especially vulnerable during the first days and weeks after LT. More than one-third of pediatric transplant recipients develop bacterial or fungal infections in the first month [55]. Careful assessment of the donor's serology and sterility analyses conducted on the graft are important. Strict hygiene measures that need to be respected by all personnel are required during the first weeks to prevent infections. Clinical and biochemical signs should be monitored closely, and adequate peri-operative antibiotic prophylaxis assured. Central venous accesses, biliary leaks and bowel perforations are the main cause for bacteremia [55]. Aggressive treatment guided by microbial identification, with appropriate antifungal prophylaxis, is key to obtain an early control of the infection. In case of mismatch between donor's and recipient's serologies for cytomegalovirus, adequate prophylaxis with specific immunoglobulins (CytoGam) should be promptly initiated within 72 h from LT to prevent the development of the disease. Long-term antifungal prophylaxis is usually required for all patients, especially when steroids are used to induce immunosuppression, and it is usually started over the first few days/weeks after transplant.

Immunosuppression and Rejection

Immunosuppression (IS) is required after LT to prevent graft rejection. Progressive discovery and implementation of new immunosuppressive regimens played a pivotal role in the improvement of graft and patient survival after LT [56]. Unfortunately, no evidence-based guidelines or consensus exist on posttransplant IS in children, and significantly different practices are observed across reference centers worldwide. All protocols are based on the principle of providing minimal levels of IS to prevent rejection while reducing toxicity. Posttransplant regimens are composed of an induction phase focused at minimizing acute rejection during the first days and weeks after LT, and a maintenance phase, which aims at inducing tolerance and reducing toxicity on the long term, while preventing acute and chronic rejection. Since T cells play a major role in acute allograft rejection, most immunosuppressive approaches are focused on them. Calcineurin inhibitors are the mainstay of treatment. Tacrolimus showed better patient and graft survival than cyclosporine, with less acute rejection, and it is now used for both induction and maintenance treatment in 95% of pediatric transplant recipients [57, 58]. A higher dose of tacrolimus is required during the first 3 months from LT. In the absence of rejection, plasma though level target is then progressively reduced, to reach maintenance levels 1 year after transplant. Nephrotoxicity is the most frequently observed side effect of tacrolimus treatment and requires close monitoring [59]. New-onset diabetes, hypertension, hyperlipidemia, and hypomagnesemia are also commonly observed. PTLD is a more rare but potentially fatal complication that requires prompt diagnosis and treatment [60]. Tacrolimus has also been associated with the development of food allergies and eosinophilic gastroenteritis in younger transplant recipients [61].

For induction, tacrolimus is most often combined with steroids (50% of pediatric LT in the U.S.) or with steroids and an antimetabolite (more frequently mycophenolate mofetil, in 25% of patients) [30]. Addition of an antimetabolite allows for reducing the dose of tacrolimus for nephroprotection. Steroid-sparing regimens with tacrolimus combined with interleukin-2 receptor antagonists (anti-CD25 antibodies, e.g. basiliximab) are increasingly used and showed improved rejection-free survival, decreased steroid-free rejection, and fewer complications [62–65]. Lymphocyte-depleting antibodies (e.g. thymoglobulin), which result in T-cell depletion and can cause significant systemic reactions, can be used instead of interleukin-2 receptor antagonists to reduce the use of steroids.

After 3 months, most patients are on a maintenance regimen, which most often is based on tacrolimus monotherapy or tacrolimus associated with an antimetabolite. Most children (75%) receive no steroids on the long term [66]. Since nonadherence is a significant cause of graft loss and late mortality in adolescence, significant effort must be dedicated to ensure proper compliance with the treatment. Extended-release tacrolimus, which allows for once-a-day dosing and proved to be comparable to standard dosing in terms of safety and efficacy, is often used in adolescents to facilitate adherence to treatment [67, 68].

Acute cellular rejection is common during the first year after LT, with reported incidence of 20–60% [30, 66]. A single episode of acute rejection was shown to have no effect on long term graft or patient survival. Rejection is more common during the first 3 months and is almost always asymptomatic, being discovered by increasing aminotransferases and GGT levels and confirmed at liver biopsy.

Intravenous administration of high-dose methylprednisolone for 1–5 days represents the first line of treatment. Subsequent tapering regimens vary widely according to the severity of the rejection, the response of the patient and institutional practice. Steroid treatment is effective in 80–90% of patients [66]. Children showing no improvement are defined as having steroid-resistant rejection and require lymphocyte-depleting antibodies, addition of mycophenolate, and maintenance of higher tacrolimus target levels for at least 3 months. Addition of mTOR inhibitors such as sirolimus can be considered in case of nonresponse.

The incidence of chronic rejection has been decreasing over the years thanks to the improvement in immunosuppressive regimens. Although biopsy-proven chronic rejection affects <10% of pediatric transplant recipients, its treatment (which consists in addressing nonadherence, increasing tacrolimus target levels, and adding mTOR inhibitors) is cumbersome and often leads to retransplantation [24, 25, 66]. Antibody-mediated rejection is an even rarer finding after liver transplantation. A well known complication after ABO-incompatible LT, it typically presents within the first 2 weeks as acute graft dysfunction often associated with fever and thrombocytopenia. Signs of acute injury with positive complement 4d staining at liver biopsy and donor-specific antibodies (DSA) are required to confirm the diagnosis [69]. Recently, antibody-mediated rejection is being increasingly detected after ABO-compatible LT, and criteria for its diagnosis are evolving [70]. Individualized treatment with corticosteroids, immunoglobulins, anti-CD20 antibodies (rituximab), plasmapheresis, or eculizumab allows for resolution of graft dysfunction in many patients.

The liver is an immunological organ, and its microenvironment has unique tolerogenic properties. Spontaneous liver allograft tolerance in animals is well described. IS withdrawal have been shown to be possible in children as in adults [71, 72]. In the largest pediatric series published by Kyoto University Hospital, 35% of LDLT patients met the criteria to withdraw IS (>2 years posttransplant, normal graft function, and no rejection over the preceding year). Of those, 44% resulted to be tolerant 1 year after withdrawal, although progressive fibrosis was often identified at biopsy and improved over reestablishment of minimal IS [73]. Data from a still unpublished prospective, multicenter, pediatric clinical trial (iWITH, NCT01638559) recently showed that 37% of the 88 patients undergoing IS withdrawal were operationally tolerant after 1 year. Interestingly, from the analysis of liver biopsies required to enter this study, the authors discovered that subclinical chronic allograft injury was indeed common even among this selected population, with almost 40% of long-term pediatric patients with normal liver tests showing liver fibrosis (Ishak stage ≥2) [74]. Although these data are encouraging and suggest that a significant proportion of patients might indeed develop tolerance over time and not need IS anymore, it is not possible yet to predict who will be tolerant upon IS withdrawal and who will end up with rejection and graft fibrosis instead. Therefore, IS withdrawal after LT is still not currently recommended.

Conclusion

Pediatric liver transplantation is now standard of care in many centers around the world. Waiting for the development of alternative cell therapy and regenerative medicine-based approaches, LT has solidly demonstrated its efficacy and overall safety across all age groups. Advancement of surgical techniques, IS regimens, and intensive care protocols led to a very significant improvement in short- and long-term graft and patient survival. Optimization of organ allocation policies to prioritize young children and reserving pediatric donors for pediatric recipients will further reduce mortality. Meanwhile, implementation and development of LDLT programs is needed to reduce the waiting time for transplant. This, together with growing surgical expertise with graft reduction, has the potential to expand the number of available organs, with the potential to virtually eliminate mortality on the wait list. Optimization of pretransplant nutritional status has emerged as a key factor to decrease posttransplant morbidity. Specialized posttransplant PICU expertise is then pivotal to allow for quick identification of posttransplant complications and improvement of pretransplant care. Studies to assess how different IS regimens can reduce long-term graft fibrosis and potential loss are warranted, while better understanding of the role of antibody-mediated rejection after LT is needed. Ongoing and future trials might lead to the identification of criteria and, ideally, biomarkers, to identify patients developing operational graft tolerance in order to program targeted IS withdrawal.

References

1. Starzl TE, Koep LJ, Schröter GP, Halgrimson CG, Porter KA, Weil R. Liver replacement for pediatric patients. Pediatrics. 1979;63:825–9.
2. Colledan M, Camagni S. In: D'Antiga L, editor. Pediatric hepatology and liver transplantation. Springer; 2019. p. 465–85. https://doi.org/10.1007/978-3-319-96400-3_27.
3. Society of Pediatric Liver Transplantation. SPLIT Registry. 2016. Accessed in March 2021 at https://splitdcc.org (data updated to September 21, 2020).
4. Mogul DB, Luo X, Bowring MG, Chow EK, Massie AB, Schwarz KB, Cameron AM, Bridges JFP, Segev DL. Fifteen-year trends in pediatric liver transplants: split, whole deceased, and living donor grafts. J Pediatrics. 2018;196:148–153.e2.
5. Kasahara M, Umeshita K, Inomata Y, Uemoto S, Society JLT. Long-term outcomes of pediatric living donor liver transplantation in Japan: an analysis of more than 2200 cases listed in the registry of the Japanese Liver Transplantation Society. Am J Transplant. 2013;13:1830–9.
6. Raia S, Nery J, Mies S. Liver transplantation from live donors. Lancet. 1989;334:497.
7. Kasahara M, Sakamoto S, Fukuda A. In: D'Antiga L, editor. Pediatric hepatology and liver transplantation; 2019. p. 487–513. https://doi.org/10.1007/978-3-319-96400-3_28.
8. Rogiers X, Malagó M, Gawad K, Jauch KW, Olausson M, Knoefel WT, Gundlach M, Bassas A, Fischer L, Sterneck M, Burdelski M, Broelsch CE. In situ splitting of cadaveric livers: the ultimate expansion of a limited donor pool. Ann Surg. 1996;224:331–41.
9. Rela M, Kaliamoorthy I, Reddy MS. Current status of auxiliary partial orthotopic liver transplantation for acute liver failure. Liver Transpl. 2016;22:1265–74.

10. Dahm F, Georgiev P, Clavien P. Small-for-size syndrome after partial liver transplantation: definition, mechanisms of disease and clinical implications. Am J Transplant. 2005;5:2605–10.
11. Urata K, Kawasaki S, Matsunami H, Hashikura Y, Ikegami T, Ishizone S, Momose Y, Komiyama A, Makuuchi M. Calculation of child and adult standard liver volume for liver transplantation. Hepatology. 1995;21:1317–21.
12. Hsu EK, Shaffer ML, Gao L, Sonnenday C, Volk ML, Bucuvalas J, Lai JC. Analysis of liver offers to pediatric candidates on the transplant wait list. Gastroenterology. 2017;153:988–95.
13. Rana A, Kueht ML, Nicholas SK, Jindra PT, Himes RW, Desai MS, Cotton RT, Galvan NTN, O'Mahony CA, Goss JA. Pediatric liver transplantation across the ABO blood group barrier: is it an obstacle in the modern era? J Am Coll Surg. 2016;222:681–9.
14. Battula NR, Platto M, Anbarasan R, Perera MTPR, Ong E, Roll GR, Neto B-HF, Mergental H, Isaac J, Muiesan P, Sharif K, Mirza DF. Intention to split policy. Ann Surg. 2017;265:1009–15.
15. Pirenne J, Monbaliu D, Gelder FV, Hees DV, Aerts R, Verslype C, Steenbergen WV, Ferdinande P, Fevery J, Nevens F, Coosemans W, Stockman W, Lormans P. Liver transplantation using livers from septuagenarian and octogenarian donors: an underused strategy to reduce mortality on the waiting list. Transplant Proc. 2005;37:1180–1.
16. Lüthold SC, Kaseje N, Jannot A, Mentha G, Majno P, Toso C, Belli DC, McLin VA, Wildhaber BE. Risk factors for early and late biliary complications in pediatric liver transplantation. Pediatr Transplant. 2014;18:822–30.
17. Spitzer AL, Lao OB, Dick AAS, Bakthavatsalam R, Halldorson JB, Yeh MM, Upton MP, Reyes JD, Perkins JD. The biopsied donor liver: incorporating macrosteatosis into high-risk donor assessment. Liver Transpl. 2010;16:874–84.
18. Everhart JE, Lombardero M, Lake JR, Wiesner RH, Zetterman RK, Hoofnagle JH. Weight change and obesity after liver transplantation: incidence and risk factors. Liver Transpl Surg. 1998;4:285–96.
19. Cuende N, Miranda B, Cañón JF, Garrido G, Matesanz R. Donor characteristics associated with liver graft survival. Transplantation. 2005;79:1445–52.
20. Kaseje N, McLin V, Toso C, Poncet A, Wildhaber BE. Donor hypernatremia before procurement and early outcomes following pediatric liver transplantation. Liver Transpl. 2015;21:1076–81.
21. Feng S, Goodrich NP, Bragg-Gresham JL, Dykstra DM, Punch JD, DebRoy MA, Greenstein SM, Merion RM. Characteristics associated with liver graft failure: the concept of a donor risk index. Am J Transplant. 2006;6:783–90.
22. Mataya L, Aronsohn A, Thistlethwaite JR, Ross LF. Decision making in liver transplantation—limited application of the liver donor risk index. Liver Transpl. 2014;20:831–7.
23. Volk ML, Goodrich N, Lai JC, Sonnenday C, Shedden K. Decision support for organ offers in liver transplantation. Liver Transpl. 2015;21:784–91.
24. Martinelli J, Habes D, Majed L, Guettier C, Gonzalès E, Linglart A, Larue C, Furlan V, Pariente D, Baujard C, Branchereau S, Gauthier F, Jacquemin E, Bernard O. Long-term outcome of liver transplantation in childhood: a study of 20-year survivors. Am J Transplant. 2018;18:1680–9.
25. Venick RS, Farmer DG, Soto JR, Vargas J, Yersiz H, Kaldas FM, Agopian VG, Hiatt JR, McDiarmid SV, Busuttil RW. One thousand pediatric liver transplants during thirty years: lessons learned. J Am Coll Surg. 2018;226:355–66.
26. Kasahara M, Umeshita K, Sakamoto S, Fukuda A, Furukawa H, Sakisaka S, Kobayashi E, Tanaka E, Inomata Y, Kawasaki S, Shimada M, Kokudo N, Egawa H, Ohdan H, Uemoto S, Society, the J. L. T. Living donor liver transplantation for biliary atresia: an analysis of 2085 cases in the registry of the Japanese Liver Transplantation Society. Am J Transplant. 2018;18:659–68.
27. Cauley RP, Vakili K, Potanos K, Fullington N, Graham DA, Finkelstein JA, Kim HB. Deceased donor liver transplantation in infants and small children: are partial grafts riskier than whole organs? Liver Transpl. 2013;19:721–9.
28. Bourdeaux C, Darwish A, Jamart J, Tri TT, Janssen M, Lerut J, Otte J-B, Sokal E, de Goyet JDV, Reding R. Living-related versus deceased donor pediatric liver transplantation: a

multivariate analysis of technical and immunological complications in 235 recipients. Am J Transplant. 2007;7:440–7.
29. Alexopoulos SP, Nekrasov V, Cao S, Groshen S, Kaur N, Genyk YS, Matsuoka L. Effects of recipient size and allograft type on pediatric liver transplantation for biliary atresia. Liver Transpl. 2017;23:221–33.
30. Kim WR, Lake JR, Smith JM, Schladt DP, Skeans MA, Noreen SM, Robinson AM, Miller E, Snyder JJ, Israni AK, Kasiske BL. OPTN/SRTR 2017 annual data report: liver. Am J Transplant. 2019;19:184–283.
31. Diamond IR, Fecteau A, Millis JM, Losanoff JE, Ng V, Anand R, Song C, Group, S. R. Impact of graft type on outcome in Pediatric liver transplantation. Ann Surg. 2007;246:301–10.
32. Darius T, Rivera J, Fusaro F, Lai Q, de Magnée C, Bourdeaux C, Janssen M, Clapuyt P, Reding R. Risk factors and surgical management of anastomotic biliary complications after pediatric liver transplantation. Liver Transpl. 2014;20:893–903.
33. Laurence JM, Sapisochin G, DeAngelis M, Seal JB, Miserachs MM, Marquez M, Zair M, Fecteau A, Jones N, Hrycko A, Avitzur Y, Ling SC, Ng V, Cattral M, Grant D, Kamath BM, Ghanekar A. Biliary complications in pediatric liver transplantation: incidence and management over a decade. Liver Transpl. 2015;21:1082–90.
34. Feier FH, Chapchap P, Pugliese R, da Fonseca EA, Carnevale FC, Moreira AM, Zurstrassen C, Santos AC, Miura IK, Baggio V, Porta A, Guimarães T, Cândido H, Benavides M, Godoy A, Leite KMR, Porta G, Kondo M, Seda-Neto J. Diagnosis and management of biliary complications in pediatric living donor liver transplant recipients. Liver Transpl. 2014;20:882–92.
35. Bekker J, Ploem S, Jong KPD. Early hepatic artery thrombosis after liver transplantation: a systematic review of the incidence, outcome and risk factors. Am J Transplant. 2009;9:746–57.
36. Ye H, Zhao Q, Wang Y, Wang D, Zheng Z, Schroder PM, Lu Y, Kong Y, Liang W, Shang Y, Guo Z, He X. Outcomes of technical variant liver transplantation versus whole liver transplantation for pediatric patients: a meta-analysis. PLoS One. 2015;10:e0138202.
37. Li J, Zu C, Li S, Gao W, Shen Z, Cai J. Effect of graft size matching on pediatric living-donor liver transplantation at a single center. Clin Transpl. 2018;32:e13160.
38. Ackermann O, Branchereau S, Franchi-Abella S, Pariente D, Chevret L, Debray D, Jacquemin E, Gauthier F, Hill C, Bernard O. The long-term outcome of hepatic artery thrombosis after liver transplantation in children: role of urgent revascularization. Am J Transplant. 2012;12:1496–503.
39. Kenari SKH, Mirzakhani H, Eslami M, Saidi RF. Current state of the art in management of vascular complications after pediatric liver transplantation. Pediatr Transplant. 2015;19:18–26.
40. Ueda M, Egawa H, Ogawa K, Uryuhara K, Fujimoto Y, Kasahara M, Ogura Y, Kozaki K, Takada Y, Tanaka K. Portal vein complications in the long-term course after pediatric living donor liver transplantation. Transplant Proc. 2005;37:1138–40.
41. de Magnée C, Bourdeaux C, Dobbeleer FD, Janssen M, Menten R, Clapuyt P, Reding R. Impact of pre-transplant liver hemodynamics and portal reconstruction techniques on post-transplant portal vein complications in pediatric liver transplantation. Ann Surg. 2011;254:55–61.
42. Alvarez F. Portal vein complications after pediatric liver transplantation. Curr Gastroenterol Rep. 2012;14:270–4.
43. de Magnée C, Veyckemans F, Pirotte T, Menten R, Dumitriu D, Clapuyt P, Carbonez K, Barrea C, Sluysmans T, Sempoux C, Leclercq I, Zech F, Stephenne X, Reding R. Liver and systemic hemodynamics in children with cirrhosis: impact on the surgical management in pediatric living donor liver transplantation. Liver Transpl. 2017;23:1440–50.
44. Herzog D, Martin SR, Lallier M, Alvarez F. Ascites after orthotopic liver transplantation in children. Pediatr Transplant. 2005;9:74–9.
45. Squires RH, Ng V, Romero R, Ekong U, Hardikar W, Emre S, Mazariegos GV. Evaluation of the pediatric patient for liver transplantation: 2014 practice guideline by the american association for the study of liver diseases, american society of transplantation and the north american society for pediatric gastroenterology, hepatolo. Hepatology. 2014;60:362–98.

46. Wiesner R, Edwards E, Freeman R, Harper A, Kim R, Kamath P, Kremers W, Lake J, Howard T, Merion RM, Wolfe RA, Krom R, Committee, T. U. N. for O. S. L. D. S. S. Model for end-stage liver disease (MELD) and allocation of donor livers. Gastroenterology. 2003;124:91–6.
47. McDiarmid SV, Anand R, Lindblad AS, Group, P. I. and I. of the S. of P. L. T. (SPLIT) R. Development of a pediatric end-stage liver disease score to predict poor outcome in children awaiting liver transplantation. Transplantation. 2002;74:173–81.
48. Bourdeaux C, Tri TT, Gras J, Sokal E, Otte J-B, de Goyet J, Reding R. PELD score and post-transplant outcome in pediatric liver transplantation: a retrospective study of 100 recipients. Transplantation. 2005;79:1273–6.
49. Hsu EK, Mazariegos GV. Global lessons in graft type and pediatric liver allocation: a path toward improving outcomes and eliminating wait-list mortality. Liver Transpl. 2017;23:86–95.
50. Swenson SM, Roberts JP, Rhee S, Perito ER. Impact of the Pediatric End-Stage Liver Disease (PELD) growth failure thresholds on mortality among pediatric liver transplant candidates. Am J Transplant. 2019;19:3308–18.
51. Carey EJ, Lai JC, Sonnenday C, Tapper EB, Tandon P, Duarte-Rojo A, Dunn MA, Tsien C, Kallwitz ER, Ng V, Dasarathy S, Kappus M, Bashir MR, Montano-Loza AJ. A North American expert opinion statement on sarcopenia in liver transplantation. Hepatology. 2019;70:1816–29.
52. Jindal A, Jagdish RK. Sarcopenia: ammonia metabolism and hepatic encephalopathy. Clin Mol Hepatol. 2019;25:270–9.
53. Córdoba J, López-Hellin J, Planas M, Sabin P, Sanpedro F, Castro F, Esteban R, Guardia J. Normal protein diet for episodic hepatic encephalopathy: results of a randomized study. J Hepatol. 2004;41:38–43.
54. Nacoti M, Cazzaniga S, Lorusso F, Naldi L, Brambillasca P, Benigni A, Corno V, Colledan M, Bonanomi E, Vedovati S, Buoro S, Falanga A, Lussana F, Barbui T, Sonzogni V. The impact of perioperative transfusion of blood products on survival after pediatric liver transplantation. Pediatr Transplant. 2012;16:357–66.
55. Shepherd RW, Turmelle Y, Nadler M, Lowell JA, Narkewicz MR, McDiarmid SV, Anand R, Song C, Group, the S. R. Risk factors for rejection and infection in pediatric liver transplantation. Am J Transplant. 2007;8:396–403.
56. Charlton MR. How important is acute cellular rejection? Liver Transpl. 2013;19:S9–S13.
57. Kelly D, Jara P, Rodeck B, Lykavieris P, Burdelski M, Becker M, Gridelli B, Boillot O, Manzanares J, Reding R. Tacrolimus and steroids versus ciclosporin microemulsion, steroids, and azathioprine in children undergoing liver transplantation: randomised European multicentre trial. Lancet. 2004;364:1054–61.
58. Kim WR, Lake JR, Smith JM, Skeans MA, Schladt DP, Edwards EB, Harper AM, Wainright JL, Snyder JJ, Israni AK, Kasiske BL. OPTN/SRTR 2015 annual data report: liver. Am J Transplant. 2017;17:174–251.
59. Kelly DA, Bucuvalas JC, Alonso EM, Karpen SJ, Allen U, Green M, Farmer D, Shemesh E, McDonald RA, Diseases, A. A. for the S. of L. & Transplantation, A. S. of. Long-term medical management of the pediatric patient after liver transplantation: 2013 practice guideline by the American Association for the Study of Liver Diseases and the American Society of Transplantation. Liver Transpl. 2013;19:798–825.
60. Marc SE, Henedina A, Claire B, Monique B, Pierre W, Ville, de G. J. de, Raymond, R., Magda, J., Paul, B. J. & Bernard, O. J. Early signs and risk factors for the increased incidence of Epstein-Barr virus-related posttransplant lymphoproliferative diseases in pediatric liver transplant recipients treated with tacrolimus. Transplantation. 1997;64:1438–42.
61. Wisniewski J, Lieberman J, Nowak-Węgrzyn A, Kerkar N, Arnon R, Iyer K, Miloh T. De novo food sensitization and eosinophilic gastrointestinal disease in children post-liver transplantation. Clin Transpl. 2012;26:E365–71.
62. Spada M, Petz W, Bertani A, Riva S, Sonzogni A, Giovannelli M, Torri E, Torre G, Colledan M, Gridelli B. Randomized trial of basiliximab induction versus steroid therapy in pediatric liver allograft recipients under tacrolimus immunosuppression. Am J Transplant. 2006;6:1913–21.

63. Reding R, Gras J, Sokal E, Otte J-B, Davies HF. Steroid-free liver transplantation in children. Lancet. 2003;362:2068–70.
64. Gras JM, Gerkens S, Beguin C, Janssen M, Smets F, Otte J-B, Sokal EM, Reding R. Steroid-free, tacrolimus-basiliximab immunosuppression in pediatric liver transplantation: clinical and pharmacoeconomic study in 50 children. Liver Transpl. 2008;14:469–77.
65. Segev DL, Sozio SM, Shin EJ, Nazarian SM, Nathan H, Thuluvath PJ, Montgomery RA, Cameron AM, Maley WR. Steroid avoidance in liver transplantation: meta-analysis and meta-regression of randomized trials. Liver Transpl. 2008;14:512–25.
66. Ng VL, Fecteau A, Shepherd R, Magee J, Bucuvalas J, Alonso E, Mcdiarmid S, Cohen G, Anand R, Group, and the S. of P. L. T. R. Outcomes of 5-year survivors of pediatric liver transplantation: report on 461 children from a North American Multicenter Registry. Pediatrics. 2008;122:e1128–35.
67. Rubik J, Debray D, Kelly D, Iserin F, Webb NJA, Czubkowski P, Vondrak K, Sellier-Leclerc A, Rivet C, Riva S, Tönshoff B, D'Antiga L, Marks SD, Reding R, Kazeem G, Undre N. Efficacy and safety of prolonged-release tacrolimus in stable pediatric allograft recipients converted from immediate-release tacrolimus – a phase 2, open-label, single-arm, one-way crossover study. Transpl Int. 2019;32:1182–93.
68. Vondrak K, Parisi F, Dhawan A, Grenda R, Webb NJA, Marks SD, Debray D, Holt RCL, Lachaux A, Kelly D, Kazeem G, Undre N. Efficacy and safety of tacrolimus in de novo pediatric transplant recipients randomized to receive immediate- or prolonged-release tacrolimus. Clin Transpl. 2019;33:e13698.
69. Demetris AJ, Bellamy C, Hübscher SG, O'Leary J, Randhawa PS, Feng S, Neil D, Colvin RB, McCaughan G, Fung JJ, Bello AD, Reinholt FP, Haga H, Adeyi O, Czaja AJ, Schiano T, Fiel MI, Smith ML, Sebagh M, Tanigawa RY, Yilmaz F, Alexander G, Baiocchi L, Balasubramanian M, Batal I, Bhan AK, Bucuvalas J, Cerski CTS, Charlotte F, Vera ME, ElMonayeri M, Fontes P, Furth EE, Gouw ASH, Hafezi-Bakhtiari S, Hart J, Honsova E, Ismail W, Itoh T, Jhala NC, Khettry U, Klintmalm GB, Knechtle S, Koshiba T, Kozlowski T, Lassman CR, Lerut J, Levitsky J, Licini L, Liotta R, Mazariegos G, Minervini MI, Misdraji J, Mohanakumar T, Mölne J, Nasser I, Neuberger J, O'Neil M, Pappo O, Petrovic L, Ruiz P, Sağol Ö, Fueyo AS, Sasatomi E, Shaked A, Shiller M, Shimizu T, Sis B, Sonzogni A, Stevenson HL, Thung SN, Tisone G, Tsamandas AC, Wernerson A, Wu T, Zeevi A, Zen Y. 2016 comprehensive update of the Banff Working Group on liver allograft pathology: introduction of antibody-mediated rejection. Am J Transplant. 2016;16:2816–35.
70. Wozniak LJ, Naini BV, Hickey MJ, Bhattacharyya S, Reed EF, Busuttil RW, Farmer DG, Vargas JH, Venick RS, McDiarmid SV. Acute antibody-mediated rejection in ABO-compatible pediatric liver transplant recipients: case series and review of the literature. Pediatr Transplant. 2017;21:e12791.
71. Bourdeaux C, Pire A, Janssen M, Stéphenne X, Smets F, Sokal EM, de Magnée C, Fusaro F, Reding R. Prope tolerance after pediatric liver transplantation. Pediatr Transplant. 2012;17:59–64.
72. Feng S, Sanchez-Fueyo A. In: D'Antiga L, editor. Pediatric hepatology and liver transplantation. Springer; 2019. p. 625–52. https://doi.org/10.1007/978-3-319-96400-3_36.
73. Ohe H, Waki K, Yoshitomi M, Morimoto T, Nafady-Hego H, Satoda N, Li Y, Zhao X, Sakaguchi S, Uemoto S, Bishop GA, Koshiba T. Factors affecting operational tolerance after pediatric living-donor liver transplantation: impact of early post-transplant events and HLA match. Transpl Int. 2012;25:97–106.
74. Feng S, Bucuvalas JC, Demetris AJ, Burrell BE, Spain KM, Kanaparthi S, Magee JC, Ikle D, Lesniak A, Lozano JJ, Alonso EM, Bray RA, Bridges NE, Doo E, Gebel HM, Gupta NA, Himes RW, Jackson AM, Lobritto SJ, Mazariegos GV, Ng VL, Rand EB, Sherker AH, Sundaram S, Turmelle YP, Sanchez-Fueyo A. Evidence of chronic allograft injury in liver biopsies from long-term pediatric recipients of liver transplants. Gastroenterology. 2018;155:1838–1851.e7.

Index

P. Jouvet, F. Alvarez (eds.), *Liver Diseases in the Pediatric Intensive Care Unit*, https://doi.org/10.1007/978-3-030-79132-2

GPSR Compliance

The European Union's (EU) General Product Safety Regulation (GPSR) is a set of rules that requires consumer products to be safe and our obligations to ensure this.

If you have any concerns about our products, you can contact us on ProductSafety@springernature.com

In case Publisher is established outside the EU, the EU authorized representative is:

Springer Nature Customer Service Center GmbH
Europaplatz 3
69115 Heidelberg, Germany

Batch number: 10732090

Printed by Printforce, the Netherlands